Marketing for health services

A framework for communications, evaluation and total quality management

Rod Sheaff

Open University Press
Milton Keynes · Philadelphia

Open University Press
Celtic Court
22 Ballmoor
Buckingham MK18 1XW

and
1900 Frost Road, Suite 101
Bristol, PA 19007, USA

First Published 1991

British Library Cataloguing in Publication Data
Sheaff, Rod
   Marketing for the NHS: a framework for communications,
   evaluation and total quality management.
   1. Great Britain. National health services. Marketing
   I. Title
   362.10688

   ISBN 0-335-15427-1 (pbk)
   ISBN 0-335-15428-X

Library of Congress Catalog number is available

Typeset by Rowland Phototypesetting Ltd
Bury St Edmunds, Suffolk
Printed in Great Britain by St Edmundsbury Press Ltd
Bury St Edmunds, Suffolk

Marketing for
health services

Contents

List of abbreviations

A&E	Accident and Emergency
ADL	Activities of Daily Living
AMSO	Association Market Survey Organisations
APACHE	Acute Physiology And Chronic Health Evaluation
ASH	Action on Smoking and Health
BMA	British Medical Association
BMRS	British Market Research Society
BSI	British Standards Institution
CASPE	Clinical Accountability Service Planning Evaluation (King's Fund)
CEO	Chief Executive Officer
CEPOD	Confidential Enquiry into Perioperative Deaths
CHC	Community Health Council
CSSD	Central Sterile Supplies Department
DGH	District General Hospital
DGM	District General Manager
DHA	District Health Authority
DMU	Directly Managed Unit
DPH	Director of Public Health
DRG	Diagnostic Related Group
ESOMR	European Society for Opinion and Market Research
FHSA	Family Health Service Authority
FOREST	Freedom Organisation for the Right to Enjoy Smoking Tobacco
GM	General Manager
HA	Health Authority
HAS	Health Advisory Service
HEA	Health Education Authority
HSE	Health and Safety Executive
IG	Income Generation
IPP	Individual Programme Planning

IPR	Individual Performance Review
LA	Local Authority
LASS	Local Authority Social Services
LEB	Life Expectancy at Birth
LMC	Local Medical Committee
LPTH	London Postgraduate Teaching Hospital
MIND	National Association of Mental Health
MRI	Manchester Royal Infirmary
NAI	Non-Accidental Injury
NAQA	National Association for Quality Assurance
NAWCH	National Association for the Welfare of Children in Hospital
NHSTA	National Health Service Training Authority
NRT	National Review Team
NWRHA	North Western Regional Health Authority
OPCS	Office of Population Census and Survey
OPD	Out-Patients Department
PAS	Patient Administration System
PIs	Performance Indicators
PST	Personal Service Team
QA	Quality Assurance
QALYs	Quality-Adjusted Life Year
QIT	Quality Improvement Team
RHA	Regional Health Authority
RMI	Resource Management Initiative
RTA	Road Traffic Accident
SGT	Self Governing Trust
SHA	Special Health Authority
SMR	Standardized Mortality Ratio
SPSS	Statistical Package for Social Scientists
SSA	Social Services Authority
SSI	Social Services Inspectorate
SWOT	Strengths, Weaknesses, Opportunities and Threats
TP	Treatment Plan
UGM	Unit General Manager
UME	United Medical Enterprises
UMIST	University of Manchester Institute of Science and Technology
UMT	Unit Management Team
USP	Unique Selling Point
WHO	World Health Organisation

Preface and Acknowledgements

This book draws upon working experience from many quarters, including activity funded by the NHS Training Authority, the King Edward Hospital Fund for London, Grimsby, Leicester, Mid Staffordshire, Parkside (London) and North Derbyshire Health Authorities. Staff in many organizations outside the NHS gave time and trouble in explaining how they address the marketing activities discussed in the text. These organizations include Black and Decker, British Airways, British Gas, British Rail, Coalite, Dunlop Tyres, the General Municipal and Boilermakers' Union, the Halifax Building Society, Holiday Inns, Jaguar Cars, London Buses, Marks and Spencer, the Metropolitan Police, Morrison Supermarkets, the National Westminster Bank, Tesco and Wood MacKenzie Retail Analysts. The text has been much improved through discussions with Peter Chisnall, Liz Fox, Roger French, Bruce Neumann, Ted O'Grady, Victor Peel, Norma Raynes, John Roberts, Angela Schofield, Michael Schofield, John Smith, Jenni Thomas and participants in the Master's course and other programmes at the Health Services Management Unit, Manchester University. If it succeeds in being a practically useful handbook much of the credit must go to Richard Baggaley.

The opinions expressed do not reflect the views of any of these organizations or individuals but are entirely the author's own, as are whatever errors remain. The illustrative vignettes are all real cases, attributed where possible but anonymized where necessary. The text concentrates on marketing for the NHS but some of the principles discussed may have wider application in other publicly-administered welfare services which are provided free at the point of use.

Denise Frost, Linda Ingle, Stephanie Mullen, Kay Stanger and Jane Silver together produced the typescript. Pauline, William and John all helped too.

Chapter 1

Marketing: the commercial prototype

Marketing reaches the NHS

Marketing is reaching the NHS. Few NHS organizations yet practice marketing consciously but many of its ingredients are already familiar to them. Among these are quality assurance, standard setting and quality circle schemes, public relations initiatives, 'personalizing' the care that NHS users receive, income generation, many patient surveys and an ill-defined but widespread interest in 'consumerism'.

One tangible sign of this is recognition in the two major health policy documents of the 1980s: Roy Griffiths's first 'report' on NHS management and *Working for Patients*. Of seven strategic objectives in the White Paper five give improved quality of patient services as their rationale and another appears to give quality of service as high a priority as achieving value for money. Two proposed mechanisms for sustaining the quality of NHS services are medical audit[1] and the 'internal' market for competition between Self Governing NHS Trusts (SGTs);

> The hospital trusts will earn revenue from the services they provide. They will therefore have an incentive to attract patients, so they will make sure that the service they offer is what patients want. And in turn they will stimulate other NHS hospitals to respond to what people want locally.[2]

Critics might dismiss this as mere rhetoric to legitimize or obscure other policy motives,[3] but there are also signs of interest in marketing in parts of the NHS far from public scrutiny, such as the annual review process. Published and teaching material on issues related to marketing is burgeoning, as are research[4] and directories of current activities[5] and research. Health Authorities are creating managerial posts with 'Quality', 'Consumer Relations', 'Public Affairs' or similar titles. Although incomplete, data on patient surveys in the period 1979–1988 collected at York University tend to confirm growth in this activity too.[6]

Although the NHS is not (yet) a conventional commercial organization, using the term 'marketing' for these areas of interest has the advantage of linking discussion of the above activities in the NHS with parallel interest in other industries: another area in which the NHS has shown increasing interest. *Working for Patients* poses the question of how the marketing in Health Authorities, self-governing trusts and directly-managed NHS services will differ from each other and from orthodox commercial marketing after 1991. Clarity on these matters is especially important for the transition period because the NHS is likely to develop a mix of non-market, 'internal' market and conventionally commercial activities all operating simultaneously. Little thought has yet been given as to whether the peculiar organizational structure of the NHS (besides its non-profit, non-market aspects) necessitates special adaptations of marketing. White paper implementation will produce yet another NHS reorganization; a rare occasion on which there is practical point in discussing not only the management of the NHS but its organizational design. It is necessary to know why marketing is relevant to the NHS if we are to understand what marketing activities the NHS might usefully adopt from other organizations, which it would need to alter and why, and which it will reject.

Explaining the relevance of marketing to current NHS objectives (beyond reorganizing itself as an 'internal market') is harder than it sounds. Marketing is only indirectly relevant to what some social theorists call the social 'function' of the NHS (whether these are taken to be the reproduction of labour power, legitimation of the social order, or whatever[7]), a function to which its managers are largely oblivious. To know these 'functions' may be indispensable to a historical or economic understanding of the NHS but hardly to its marketing. The report of the Royal Commission on the NHS was the nearest the NHS has so far come to producing an explicit, formal and public code of objectives. It lists NHS objectives as being to:

1 Encourage and assist individuals to remain healthy
2 Ensure equal entitlement to services
3 Provide a broad range of services of high standard
4 Ensure equal access to these services
5 Provide health care free at time of use
6 Satisfy reasonable public expectations for health care
7 Provide a national service responsive to local needs[8]

Working for Patients reiterates items 3, 5, 6 and 7.

Two other main current objectives of the NHS are to provide community care where possible for the elderly infirm, the mentally ill and the mentally and physically handicapped; and to minimize the public cost of the NHS as part of a wider strategy for reducing the state sector in the UK economy. The former objective is of course formulated above all in the second Griffiths report *Community Care; Agenda for Action*.[9] Whilst the latter is publicly recognized by government it is certainly not proclaimed as loudly as the claims that government now spends more on the NHS than ever before. However, its importance in practice is revealed by the priorities and foci of attention of NHS managerial processes, for instance the weight attached to the Resource Management Initiatives.

To these objectives can be added those that the NHS arguably ought also to adopt, above all the WHO policy of *Health for All 2000*. Its European Regional targets include 'resources distributed according to need' and 'effective mechanisms for ensuring quality of patient care'[10] but the majority recommend maintenance of health and prevention of sickness through influencing personal health behaviours (e.g. diet, stress management) and occupational health care, intersectoral activities to reduce environmental hazards and accidents, and provision of adequate housing, water and sanitation besides tackling major preventable causes of death such as heart disease.[11] NHS health promoters are already aware of the practical usefulness of marketing methods.

Insofar as a single objective dominated debates over creating the NHS, it was providing health services for 100% of the population when required, wherever and in whatever form required[12] without commercial or financial barriers.[13] Even the prime minister's foreword to *Working for Patients* endorses this.[14] Once *Working for Patients* is implemented it is the buyers who will inherit these objectives about needs and it will fall to the buyers to articulate user needs and wishes into contractual terms. Once formal and financial barriers to access to health care have been removed, class, racial and other social differences in service uptake become attributable not to better health status (because *ceteris paribus* the classes lower down the social scale tend to have a lower health status[15] but to such factors as attitudes to health–care professionals, self-image, attitudes and habits in self–care and material life-style. These are precisely the sort of areas which organizations outside the NHS have long used marketing methods to influence.

The possible contribution of marketing to the objective of meeting patient needs is important for another reason. A strong ethical case can be made for taking the meeting of patient needs as the fundamental criterion by which the provision of health care is justified, and therefore by which to judge health care organizations and the health system itself. These arguments on the basis of need apply to every potential patient (and some would argue, simply to every human[16]) whereas arguments based on NHS objectives apply to NHS managers and staff by virtue only of their official and professional capacities. If marketing assisted health services in meeting user needs, the ethical point alone would be a conclusive argument for the relevance of marketing to health services. Because the concept of 'need' is more complex than it first appears, and because the main concern of this work is marketing not ethics, the ethical dimension is only mentioned here, for the sake of completeness. It has been amply discussed elsewhere.[17] Analogous ethical arguments apply to ensuring high quality care and to preventing ill health.[18]

In implementing community care, marketing can offer health managers the framework and techniques for recruiting the support of informal carers, local authority planners besides those NHS staff who have become as dependent on the long-stay institutions as their residents (Vignette 2 illustrates this). The marketing method of 'segmenting' (explained below) can be used as a vehicle for positive discrimination and for tailoring service design more closely to the needs of the clients themselves.

Since the 1976 financial crisis, cost containment has become an increasingly central objective in health policy. But (unless the underlying objective is simply to discredit the public provision of health services) a cheaper service is of little use if no one wants to use it or its quality is unnecessarily low,[19] marketing methods can at least limit this damage. Pressure to contain costs is likely to continue for economic reasons largely extraneous to health policy, and irrespective of which parliamentary party is in office. Implementation of *Working for Patients* is likely to transmit these financial pressures also onto GP medical services, hitherto comparatively protected from them. In response it is open to the NHS to respond to pursue its claims for further resources, and indeed its other health policy objectives such as the reduction of alcohol abuse, through public debate and through the political arena: in short, through the techniques of 'social marketing'.[20]

In the 1970s re-emergent 'consumerist' and politically radical organizations began to place new demands on the NHS. Feminists were especially active, raising demands about abortion and forms of childbirth. As a token CHCs were tagged on to the new managerial structures in 1974. The Royal Commission accepted that NHS objectives ought to include responsiveness to users' demands, or at least to 'reasonable' ones. Roy Griffiths' Report recommended NHS managers to;

> ascertain how well the service is being delivered at local level by obtaining the experience and perceptions of patients and the community: these can be derived from CHCs and by other methods, including market research and from the experience of general practice and the community health services; . . . respond directly to this information; . . . act on it in formulating policy; . . . monitor performance against it; . . . promote realistic public and professional perceptions of what the NHS can and should provide as the best possible service within the resources available.[21]

More concretely, *Working for Patients* recommends reliable appointments systems, more pleasant waiting facilities, clearer information and suggestions systems and 'optional extras and amenities' in hospitals, implicitly on the grounds that this is what the public demands.[22] Marketing is also potentially relevant to the NHS as a method for identifying user demands systematically and responding practically.

The possibility of contributing to these objectives makes marketing worth considering for NHS use. The next sections outline the commercial, prototype forms of marketing. Chapter 2 then considers whether this prototype can, or should be, applied to the NHS and if so, with what modifications. Chapters 3 to 6 then explain the practicalities of the model of NHS marketing that results.

Marketing policy and objectives

Business planning

The rest of this chapter outlines a generic model of commercial marketing, which many texts elaborate more fully.[23] In practice different firms concentrate upon, and perform most successfully, different aspects of the generic model of commercial marketing.

Marketing objectives in a commercial setting derive from the firm's corporate objectives. These are 'structural' objectives in the sense of being determined by the firm's inherent characteristics as a profit-maximizer in a competitive market and as a capital with shareholders and employees. Examination of how marketing objectives derive from corporate objectives illustrates how marketing contributes to achieving the firm's overall objectives and how some characteristics of marketing derive from the commercial use of marketing rather than being inherent in the process of product design, promotion and so on which are outlined below.

Firms' main objectives are formulated in their business plans. The format of the business plan is usually individual to the firm writing it. Because of their potential value to competitors these plans are highly confidential. Nevertheless some tentative generalizations are possible.

The overall commercial objectives and goals of most would probably include objectives and goals formulated in terms of net profit (many firms differentiate profit 'optimization' from short-run 'maximization'), profit growth, return on investment, dividend per share, profit per employee, profit return on sales, sales figures (in cash and in volume terms) and market shares. Exact definitions and interpretations of these indicators (and of others like them) differ from firm to firm. Nevertheless they all are specifiable, indeed quantifiable. (For instance market share would be stated as a percentage of a known or estimated market size, not verbally as 'big' or 'bigger'.) Timescales for planning will also vary from firm to firm but are often in the order of three to five, sometimes ten years.

Publics

Commercial objectives determine who the firm's main 'publics' are and their order of importance. (Confusingly these publics are also referred to as 'customers' in some cases.) Of these, the shareholder is clearly first. Not that this makes shareholders the public that commercial marketers will usually make the most effort to influence; in most circumstances the shareholders do not have to be induced to change their behaviours or motivations, to meet the firm's commercial objectives more effectively. (For many firms, including recently privatized ones such as British Gas, the great majority of shares (some 80% in the case of British Gas) are owned by institutions not individuals.) However there are exceptions, for instance when takeover looms and during the mandatory reporting to shareholders. These occasions are not typical of most marketing activity and shareholders are not usually the recipient of the bulk of the marketing attention.

Potential and existing customers are the 'public' who, for obvious reasons, receive the bulk of marketing attention. As shown below, this 'public' may comprise of many distinct markets and market segments. Here 'customer' may not necessarily mean the end user of the product. Nowadays this is commonly the case only in retailing, transport, catering, finance and other service industries. Wholesalers, brokers or retailers who actually sell the product or service are of course such an important public that a large proportion of promotional activity will often be targeted specifically at them. The rest of this chapter concentrates mainly on how this customer public is addressed.

Many firms also develop goals for their relations with other, subordinate 'publics'. These might include such goals as projecting an image of being a technical innovator, industry leader (e.g. IBM) or responsive and caring about staff, consumers and community (e.g. Marks and Spencer).

Within the firm, staff are a major public. This is especially so in service industries because the 'product' largely consists of a social interaction between staff and customers (e.g. in retailing or banking). It can equally be important where there are industrial relations problems (e.g. in the case of Dunlop around the time of its takeover by Sumitomo) and when the firm depends critically on one group of staff (e.g. sales staff in retailing). Other parts of the vertical 'chain' of production are also an important public. Building a close relationship with suppliers (as, for instance, Marks and Spencer try to do) makes it easier to manage the quality of the products finally offered for sale.

Government is also an important public, not only as a major customer for many firms (e.g. for Ferranti and other weapons makers), but because of their ability to influence unilaterally the legal and regulatory climate in which the firm trades. (Recently the brewers have had to pay attention to this 'public'.) As one means to influence 'public' opinion and government, the mass media are a third important public for many firms, especially those whose standing in public esteem is precarious (e.g. the tobacco industry) or those such as banks for whom customers' 'confidence' is necessary for successful trading. Charitable giving to popular causes (health care not the least) can also enable firms to improve their public image. However the benefits can also be more direct. In choosing which hospitals or school to donate to, many US firms will select those used by their staff and staff dependants, thereby addressing two publics at once.

Consumer groups can from time to time be either an important public, or a public relations problem for firms and hence another important public, whether because of their possible influence on government or the media or because of a direct influence on sales. Examples might include CAMRA, the environmental groups such as Greenpeace towards which ICI and other oil and chemical makers appear to be becoming increasingly sensitive and the groups of thalidomide victims and their relatives campaigning against the Distillers' company.

A review of objectives and of definitions of who the main 'publics' are sometimes leads a to redefinition of key business; e.g. 1985 US Holiday Inns redefined its core business and accordingly renamed itself as Holiday Corporation because it was approaching saturation of its traditional markets.[24]

Redefinitions of the key business is more than a cosmetic matter of image because it can indicate complete reorientation of the business activity towards new sets of markets. Together the commercial objectives, the selection of the firm's major 'publics', and the relative emphases attached to different objectives and publics constitute the firm's business strategy. One manifestation of the attempt to define the key business orientation, as well as the firm's main objectives, is the production of the 'mission statement' or 'philosophy' discussed below.

Market strategies

Because the firms objectives are achieved by using the market, the derivation of its marketing objectives is usually mediated by (firstly) an analysis of what market types each main market is and (secondly) an audit of the firm's and its competitors' current marketing activity in each of these markets (i.e. a 'marketing audit').[25] All this is done with an eye to the state of the industry as a whole at its markets, of competitors and of the wider economic and social environment.

Several standard managerial grids already exist for the analysis of market types once the firm has enumerated its main intended markets. Individual firms in practice adapt these grids to their own use, adding or substituting other criteria of their own in making the strategic marketing decisions about which markets to compete in. Marks and Spencer, for instance, also want to be seen as a respectable, responsible firm which does not lure its customers into excessive debt and this consideration has influenced their decision as to whether to compete in the 'shop card' credit arena. One grid is outlined here to give the reader unfamiliar with commercial marketing a flavour of the sorts of strategic decisions that have to be made. Fuller details are in the texts cited.

The Boston Consulting Group matrix is perhaps the best known, according to which there are four main product and market types. 'Star' products have high market share in a high-growth market and therefore merit a high level of marketing support to sustain their sales growth. 'Cash cow' products have a high market share but low sales growth prospects. A lower level of marketing support will ordinarily be necessary here, mainly with the view to defending market share. 'Problem child' or 'question mark' products have low market shares in a high-growth market. With these the strategic marketing decision is whether they have potential to become a 'star' and accordingly ought to be given marketing support or ought to be abandoned. 'Dogs' are products with low shares of a slow-growing market. The merits of giving these large-scale marketing support are even more questionable.[26]

Alternative grids include Igor Ansoff's product opportunity matrix[27], the Profit Impact of Marketing Strategy[28], the General Electric Business Screen[29], and Porter's Generic Strategy Model.[30] Because of its applicability to the US health system, it is also worth mentioning the grid developed by Kotler and Clarke[31] which, with the other grids, is outlined in Chapter 3.

These grids (and the other methods which are used to analyse market types) guide the decision about which markets the firm should concentrate on for profit maximization, and provide very broad outlines of marketing strategy for each market. Each grid conceptualizes and recommends different market 'positions' for firms in different commercial circumstances. Bearing in mind the commercial objectives and priorities among the various 'publics' this outline is then translated into a marketing strategy. Seldom, if ever, are business objectives translated simply and directly into marketing objectives. The firm's global objectives also have to be translated into financial, production and other objectives and the resulting sets of objectives all made consistent with one another and with the marketing objectives. More important than this is the necessity to specify and work up the firm's marketing strategy through a process of marketing audit of each market.

Marketing audit

The results of a marketing audit can be summarized in the so called 'SWOT' ('strengths, weaknesses, opportunities and threats') analysis. A marketing audit consists of a detailed account of all the factors influencing a market. From it can be made a comparison of the firm's own marketing with its competitors' marketing strategy.

Among the items considered in detail are product specifications and quality, including supplier, cost and technical limitations on the product or service that can be provided. Product research and development has also to be considered. The firm's public image and the impact of its advertising, can be analysed, the strengths and weaknesses of the salesforce, retail outlets used and their characteristics. Profiles of existing customers examine who the customers are, the product range they require, and their demands in terms of product quality, cost and availability. Market opportunities and the relationships between price, quality, volume of sales and discounts are also considered.

Marketing audits also audit who the main competitors are, their intentions and ability to compete. This is particularly important for markets due to be deregulated. In the middle 1980s, for instance, building societies and the banks were both trying to assess how to defend their traditional markets against the other group of institutions and how to diversify into markets previously reserved for the other type of financial organization.

Explicit assumptions are also formulated about the state of markets and economic and social trends which influence consumption patterns. Over the past decade the increased numbers of working women would be one such factor in consumer goods markets, as (more recently) is increased public consciousness of 'green' issues. Marks and Spencer, on the other hand, became increasingly aware of a slowdown in growth in its traditional main markets. Attempts are often made to anticipate (or influence) fashions, for instance the colour or 'look' of products or the recycling of 'youth cultures'. This can extend to health issues; some supermarkets have anticipated the possibility of charging premium prices for 'organic' food, fruit or vegetables, and many food manufacturers try to associate their products with images of health or fitness.

It is taken as sound commercial practice to make the assumptions and data of the marketing audit, and the resulting strategy, clear and explicit so that they can be corrected if necessary as markets change. The firm's business strategy, choice of markets and marketing strategy also imply the acceptable levels of risk and for investment in new products, and hence the overall budgets for marketing and the managerial control indicators for it (e.g. indicators such as the minimum acceptable ratio of sales yielded to marketing costs).

From these considerations and from its marketing audit, a firm can produce its marketing plan. The latter specifies exactly which marketing techniques are to be used, and in what ways, to implement the marketing strategy. Undertaking a marketing audit, finalizing a marketing strategy and producing a marketing plan requires market research. The next task is to outline the contribution of market research to these activities.

Assessing consumer demands through market research

Consumers and consumption

Market research in a commercial setting is essentially applied research into how markets can be used to further the firm's main objectives, central among which is profitability.[32] Market research occurs only as a means to achieve these objectives but this alone makes it a central managerial activity for commercial organizations. Interested readers are referred to the many text-books on the technicalities of commercial market research.[33]

Two main elements have to be researched. First, is the attempt to forecast effective demand. Whilst sales forecasts are central to this they are of limited use without an understanding of what influences sales; more on this shortly. Secondly, it is necessary to consider how the firm can maximize the demand it faces by practically influencing those influences upon sales which it can. What the firm can influence is a 'marketing mix' of components of its own marketing strategy, explained in the next section. Market research is therefore primarily a support tool for decision making on such matters.

To discover the scale of potential demand and what influences it, commercial market research focuses upon the buying decision and what influences that. In consumer-goods markets this generally places the focus upon the consumer's characteristics. (Generally but not always: decisions to buy baby food for instance are made by adults.) Following the commoner case we shall here treat the consumer as the buyer.

The consumer himself or herself is the first item researched. In commerce it is especially important to establish what motivates them to buy. Market researchers commonly investigate the main consumer groups' occupation, their income where possible (consumers are often reluctant to disclose it), their geographic distribution, age, sex, stage in the life cycle and other social characteristics. Because products are increasingly purchased for psychological reasons (as well as for sheer functionality) it is important for marketers to know what symbols and values the buyer attaches to the product (e.g. whether furniture is being purchased to display the buyer's taste or his wealth). The reason why some buyers are loyal to a particular brand[34], and what differentiates people with a large, regular consumption of a given product from occasional consumers is also a favourite topic for market research.

Consumer psychology has attracted special interest and a mass of secondary research can be brought to bear upon such matters as consumers' behaviour, their motivation, their perceptual processes, their character traits, 'psychographics' of their attitudes and the influences which their social 'reference groups' have upon them.[35] Further research has accumulated around methods of classifying the different types of benefit consumers expect from a given product.[36] These methods have proved to be of varying usefulness to marketers in practice.

A corollary is market research into consumption patterns, investigating the uses to which the consumer puts the product (e.g. whether a particular model of car is bought mainly for fleets, for family use, etc.), how, when, where and why the product is consumed (e.g. whether fast food is bought by parents or by children, as a treat or as stopgap when nothing else can be had, etc.). This suggests what products are seen by the consumer as substitutes and complements to the product. For example most spending on DIY goods occurs within a year of moving, suggesting that furniture might be a complementary line for DIY retailers to expand into. Such techniques as brand mapping are used to explore what characteristics the consumer attributes to the product and the features by which he or she differentiates this product from others. It is important to know who makes the decision to buy. For example in the 1950s buying decisions abouts men's clothes were more often made by mothers and wives than they now are. This change has had obvious implications for the targeting of adverts and the messages to be conveyed, and less obvious implications about the design, packaging and merchandising of clothes. Knowledge of the buying process from initial need-arousal to the post-purchase evaluation of the goods is another favourite marketing research theme.

New customers can be attracted partly by 'selling to' the strengths which consumers believe a product to have (e.g. safety in the case of Volvo cars) or by cultivating ability to sell a product tailored to the demands of a distinct customer segment ('niche marketing') as, say, Rolls Royce cars do. Since advertising and other forms of promotion are believed to play a large part in retaining customer loyalty and attracting new custom, one common line of market research is to consider the impact of advertisements, whether they convey the intended messages and how long their impact lasts. To supplement this much secondary research on communications theory, perception and semiotics are available.[37]

Whole new markets, however, can only arise if the firm can find market gaps where a potentially profitable demand exists for a product which is not yet being supplied. A major use of market research is to detect such opportunities. If a possible market gap is found, market research is used at three stages in product development to check whether the new product is likely to fill the gap profitably. 'Concept testing' tries to discover before the product or service is actually provided how the consumer is likely to react. For example one firm recently conducted market research to discover how consumers might react to the idea of paying £5.00 for a personalized greetings card for the one or two people closest to them. If this proves promising the next major stage is to test a prototype product experimentally. If this proves successful, 'test marketing' can be undertaken to find the price at which it can be sold and the most effective channels for distributing it. Marks and Spencer have used this approach in introducing new product lines in clothing and furniture.

Competitors

Opportunities to sell are of course limited by competitors' activities. Another main use of commercial market research is to assess the firm's strengths and weaknesses against its competitors. A first problem is to define who the competitors are; they include not only sellers of a very similar product (so for example a European airline would probably wish to research the marketing strengths and weaknesses of other European airlines) but producers of substitute products (in this case our airline might also wish to research the marketing position of express train services as a main competitor on short-haul routes). The analysis extends beyond the product and service offered towards such factors as the image of the firm, its rivals and their products. This might include such factors as which firm customers regard as the market leader, how far they recognize and recall the competing brand names, what image and how stable customer loyalty to each brand or firm is.

Environmental changes also influence selling opportunities and market research will therefore often cover technological developments and changes in social habits. For instance the gradual increase in divorce is seen by at least one car manufacturer as creating potential new markets for cars as the one-car family disintegrates into two car-owning individuals. Lastly the legal and regulatory framework has also to be reviewed. In Europe trade liberalization and the creation of a common European market in 1992 has made this aspect of market research important recently. One major European airline laid its plans for the common European market as early as 1987.

Vignette 1.1 illustrates the range of questions investigated by one building society's market research activity recently.

Such multidimensional data require a correspondingly wide set of data collection methods, drawn from a wide range of social and natural sciences. Quantitative data required for these methods can be obtained partly from routine administrative and financial sources, in particular the analysis of invoices and credit applications. What attracted Marks and Spencer to introducing a charge card (for instance) was the possibility of using the data so collected for targeted direct mailings and promotions. Questionnaires, complaint analysis (e.g. product returns) and opinion polling are commonly used. Qualitative data can be obtained through such media as focus groups, one-to-one interviews, interpretative psychological tests, analysis of media coverage and the testing of competitors' products. Japanese motor manufacturers are known to buy large numbers of the cars against which their product will be competing and to dismantle and test these exhaustively.

Vignette 1.1   The architecture of market research

The Halifax is the largest building society in Britain with over 11 million customers and branches in virtually every town. The new Building Societies Act and the deregulation of financial markets motivated it to its first use of competition surveys, including scrutiny of comparable US institutions, and to expand its central marketing services department. Market research was undertaken on:

- Corporate image
- Product offering image
- Customers' preferred methods of funding and paying for purchases
- Attitudes to cash dispensers
- Images of different ways of saving and investing
- Awareness and views of different organizations offering financial services especially direct competitors
- Image of financial organizations
- Customer attitudes of financial management, stocks and shares
- Impression given by advertisements and viewers' recall of them
- 24-hour services
- One-stop shopping
- Efficiency of house purchasing processes (e.g. copy of valuations, confirmation of availability of mortgage).

Both qualitative and quantitative researches were made, using a panoply of methods. Three examples are:

1 Focus group discussions of six–ten people who have been matched for age, income and interests. The group is led by a facilitator, often experienced in psychological techniques, and used to gain an in-depth understanding of motives, feelings and values *vis-à-vis* a particular subject area.

2 Telephone surveys simply let the Halifax cover more people in a given period

of time with fewer questioners. It has been found that some people are more forthcoming because of the anonymity.

3 Initial questionnaires are formulated to establish attitudes, perceptions and key variables in terms of the intended target market and the intended offering to that target market. For instance, because of Building Societies' current image, their customers expect more comprehensible products geared towards the 'average man or woman' rather than the financial connoisseurs. So although the Halifax might offer stocks and shares, they must be offered in such a way as to not intimidate customers. The initial questionnaires need to test the assumptions about who might want them, in what form, how, where and at what cost so that profiles can be built up of target customers, desired product range, environment and service needs, and to what extent the Halifax fits potential customers' expectations.

The degree of specificity sought by Halifax's market research is illustrated by these examples:

1 A recent exercise to look at a proposed 'contents only' insurance policy used groups fulfilling the following criteria:

(i) All members were the main financial decision maker for a household;
(ii) At least half were Halifax customers;
(iii) All were either home owners or long-standing tenants;
(iv) All had taken out or renewed their home contents policies within the last six months.

2 Halifax wanted to check that their Cardcash television advertising was successful and it was therefore necessary to assess its effectiveness in terms of its ability to communicate the desired information about the Cardcash account and its ability to reach the target market: viewers who would be interested in opening a Cardcash account. They therefore used Granada Televisions's 'Talkback' service. This lets a subscriber measure the reaction of a panel of television viewers to a commercial after seeing it on their own TV set. Responses are sent immediately via the telephone lines to a computer for analysis. For the study of the Halifax's Cardcash commercial questions ranged from general about the account to specifics on such features as bill paying and interest. They checked which messages within the commercial were memorable and how viewers thought the Halifax commercial compared with those from other Building Societies. They also asked whether the viewers would open a Cardcash account and their reasons for doing so. Analysing the answers by the viewers' socio-demographic characteristics produced a detailed interpretation of the advert's effect.

All this is supplemented from two secondary sources. One is published material on predicted growth in particular sectors of the economy, and demographic projections of the changes in sizes of occupational groups and so on. For obvious reasons recent market research which might be of competitive use is kept confidential and without resorting to industrial espionage little help is usually available from this source. However, commercial databases collect data of common interest to all firms in an industry and sell it to subscribers who then interpret for themselves and augment it with data confidential to themselves. Their market research methods often include consumer panels and statistical sampling of retailers. Marketing research provides the other secondary source. A hint of its range and complexity is given above.

Analysis and segmentation

The resulting data has then to be analysed. Again methods taken from academic work in natural and social sciences are applied or adapted. In a commercial setting where there is not always the money, the need, nor above all the time, to do research to the highest academic or scientific standards, a

---

Vignette 1.2   Railway segmentation

British Rail's *Quality Assurance Monitor* illustrates how to analyse and present market research data. Produced by outside consultants, it is distributed under the imprint of the BR Board. A management summary at the outset of each issue outlines the main improvements and deteriorations in BR's performance in its main markets. Later analysis expands these points for the main areas of managerial concern. 'Customer perceptions' and 'Performance against corporate plan objectives' (for the current year) mainly concern passenger services. Further analyses cover freight and parcels services. Each heading presents a mixture of data, drawn from a variety of internal and external sources.

British Rail has for many years been defending its market share against newer forms of transport (car, air) and lately against deregulated markets (buses, air shuttles). For this reason market research has long concentrated on Intercity services.

The research revealed two main categories of passenger. At one extreme were business travellers, concerned with speed and punctuality. Provided fares were broadly competitive with short-haul airlines these customers were not unduly influenced by fare levels because the employer would normally pay. For the same reason their demand for food on trains was for meals broadly at restaurant standards and prices. Around London, crowding on peak-hour trains remains a concern.

At the opposite extreme were leisure travellers for whom fare levels were a more important consideration because they met the cost themselves; hence the variety of Saver and railcard tickets. Less experienced travellers than the business clientele, their main concerns included problems of changing trains, whether children would enjoy the journey and the availability of light, comparatively cheap snacks.

This sort of information made it possible to design the presentation of train services for the different segments within the Intercity sector. Analogous methods are used within the other customer sectors; freight, parcels, London commuters, provincial passengers and Railfreight. British Rail have also used segmentation to discriminate markets in which they do not wish to operate. Railfreight, for instance, has focussed on whole train-loads of single commodities and containers. Small, mixed-short-distance freight work is not so actively sought. The opening of the Channel tunnel and the increasing use of 'just in time' manufacturing present the possibility of new segments to exploit.

method of 'triangulation' is often used to cross check the different data sources. Similarly, market research is sometimes undertaken at two levels. First a comparatively broad overview of consumers, competitors, markets and environment is used for issue identification, to discover where it is likely to be worthwhile concentrating the marketing effort. Then, in these areas, more detailed and quantitative research is applied so that market research expertise is concentrated on the decisions committing the largest sums of money.

A major concern in the analysis is to identify distinct 'segments' among the customers. Its essence is to identify empirically sub-populations among the clientele whose demand patterns are so distinct as to require their own product range.[38] Vignette 1.2 illustrates this. British Gas segments its customers as 'domestic', 'commercial' and 'industrial'.

Segmentation offers four advantages. Firstly, a firm may achieve higher sales, turnover and profit by offering each segment a product tailored for it than by selling a standard product to all. Secondly, segmentation can be used to pre-empt competition. For example, some manufacturers sell their product for retailers to package and sell as an 'own brand' in competition with the manufacturer's own brand name. Perverse though this seems, the manufacturer prefers it to another supplier competing.[39] Thirdly, segmentation can be used to discriminate profitable, potentially profitable and unprofitable customer groups. British Rail, for instance, long since decided by this method not to compete in the markets for transporting livestock or small local freight consignments. Lastly, segmentation lets the firm's line-management hierarchies correspond to the main customer segments, making one manager uniquely responsible for serving that segment. If this arrangement is superimposed over other management structures a matrix organization results. British Rail, for example, operated from 1948 with a regional managerial structure, on which it later imposed a structure corresponding to its main customer segments (Intercity, Railfreight, etc.) Such an approach implies the necessity for reorganization following any radical change in customer segmentation.

Analysis of market research data usually involves comparison with three main bench marks. The first is the firm's own performance in the recent past in terms of (for example) sales, market share, numbers of complaints, etc. Second is the equivalent performance of rivals and in particular whether these are gaining or losing ground. Both these analyses require data to be collected regularly and often so that trends can be detected. Exactly how often depends on the nature of the product, the competitiveness of the market and the resources of the firm. However it is not uncommon for quantitive data to be analysed quarterly and more often for key data such as sales and turnover, with a broader and more thorough review every one or two years. The third benchmark is the firm's stated objectives themselves. Market research thus provides a major monitoring tool as well as a decision support tool.

Such extensive, frequent data collection and analysis requires considerable resourcing, and skilled market researchers command salaries on a level with senior managers. Although it may often be cheaper to sub-contract market research than to do it in-house considerable sums of money may be involved. For example an opinion poll from a reputable supplier will have a start-up cost in the order of £1000 and additional costs of £200 or more per question to a sample of 1000 people. Marketing consultancy will ordinarily cost in the range £200 to £1000 per consultant-day. To reduce these costs industry-wide marketing databases exist, for instance in pharmaceutical and supermarket retailing.

This market research is used to finalize the firm's marketing strategy and decide the consequent marketing mix. The next section explores this.

Producing a marketing mix

Products

A commercial marketing mix is produced by adjusting the firm's main marketing tools' in the way market research suggests will maximise demands, sales and profits. McCarthy famously categorized marketing tools under the headings product, price, promotion, place.[40] Since his classification is popular among both practitioners and students we will follow it here in illustrating the main components of a marketing mix.

The marketing mix produced by using these tools is manifested in the firm's operational policies and in designing and providing products or services to satisfy effective demand. Market research also reveals any segmentation of the firm's markets, the benefits different segments seek from the products and any potentially profitable gaps in the market. The marketing tools have to be applied differently in each segment, but also in a mutually compatible way both within and between segments so that the different tools reinforce one another's effects.[41]

Product decisions are McCarthy's first element in a marketing mix. At the outset product mix has to be decided: which products are to be produced and which emphasized in implementing the marketing plan. Profitability can only be achieved in the long run by ensuring that the product mix includes products at different stages in the product life cycle. Figure 1.1 illustrates how sales, income and profit will typically flow during this life cycle, and the usual distribution of marketing costs. (The exact shape of the product life cycle curves for seasonal products, fads and certain other product types varies from that shown but the four stages outlined below are common.)

In the innovation phase prototype products are developed, tested and technically perfected. Naturally this stage tends to be the most commercially sensitive and secretive but it is for example known at the time of writing that a Japanese car maker is at this stage in developing products for the European 'executive car' market. Marketing costs here arise from concept and product testing. Diffusion begins when the product has been prepared for the market and can be sold on an increasing scale as it wins acceptability, as competitiors produce a similar product, and as it becomes possible to reduce prices and

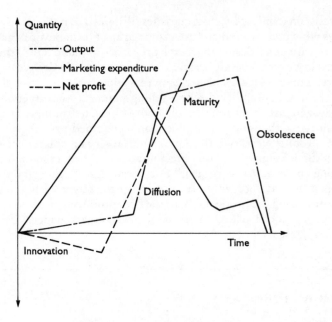

Figure I.I Product life cycle

increase the scale of production. In these stages there is a very high rate of product failure. It has been estimated that in the US only 20% of new product ideas survive the innovation phase and the first year of the dissemination phase, and only 10% earn a 'satisfactory return'.[42] There are high marketing costs in launching a product and establishing a (new) market for it.

When the market is saturated the stage of maturity is reached. Sales continue on a replacement basis and perhaps display a slower rate of growth reflecting underlying growth in the population and in the economy. Marketing can fall back to the level necessary to maintain brand loyalty once the stage of maturity is reached. Obsolescence sets in as a replacement product enters its diffusion phase. The replacement may be a technical replacement (e.g. microchips instead of transistors) or a purely stylistic replacement (e.g. when free-standing ovens are replaced with a functionally identical kitchen-unit mounted oven). Then there may be a last burst of promotional activity as attempts are made to sell off the last nearly-obsolete products before the replacements dominate the market.

With suitable market research available on the benefits users seek from the product, consumer profiles and consumption patterns, the product can be designed to anticipate and meet consumer demand. Design takes place on two main levels; functional and cultural. In a commercial setting both aspects are usually specified on the basis of market research findings.

Functional design concerns the technical characteristics of the product. In the case of cars this would include such attributes as engine specification, wind resistance and safety characteristics. Provided that the technical characteristics which buyers demand are provided at a profitable price and production cost, functional design is generally regarded as the sphere of the technical expert. However there are exceptions, one being the designed life of the product. This is often a balance between opposing promotional considerations. Product durability can be a selling point (cf. the advertisement line 'Volkswagen cars – very tough as old boots') and it may not profit a firm to let its products be thought less durable than its competitors'. Against this, the sooner a product wears out, the quicker and larger can replacement sales be.[43]

Cultural design is of more direct interest to the marketers. It consists in designing the product to be 'read' as a social sign. Such a sign can convey many messages at once: about the self-image the buyer wishes to project by buying and using the product, about the firm producing it, about the buyer's life-style and social place. Many of these signs are widely and instantly recognizable (see Vignette 1.3).

Vignette 1.3   Road signs

Car enthusiasts give great weight to the technical performance and specification of the cars they buy. These buyers, however, are exceptional. Most buyers choose their cars largely on the cars' 'marketing mix' characteristics. Price and the sheer availability of a suitable model are obviously important factors. But scarcely less important for the buyers of new cars especially is the way in which the car can act as, among other things, a social sign of the driver's tastes and of the impression of his or her personality and social place that he or she wishes to project. This is fairly obvious in the case of Rolls Royce, Porsche or the 'executive car' market, in which the sheer costliness of the car can be a selling point. However, less expensive cars are also used and seen as social signs in this way. A recent article in *Today* illustrates how widely these signs are understood. About various cars the journalist comments:

> Women who play safe in life pick a Fiesta to play safe on the roads . . .

> Apart from economy and safety these people (Peugeot 205 owners) want a car that projects a trendy image and gets them to important meetings on time . . .

> The man or woman who drives a BMW 3 series has made it in life and likes everyone to know it. They think the car suits their image, which they see as sophisticated and tasteful.

> Renault 5 drivers keep their car immaculately tidy and take great pride in keeping it shiny. Appearances are very important to them.

All these are just one journalist's interpretations of how cars act as a social 'sign'. Nevertheless the ways in which the buying public 'read' (or misread) these signs are in a commercial setting of great importance to salesforces, advertisers and product designers.

Source: Moore, J., 'Car Gazing' *Today* 30th March 1989.

These signs work not only at the conscious level; much marketing and psychological research has explored the implicit and unconscious ways in which products are also designed, bought and consumed as social signs.[44]

The more functionally similar mass-produced products in a given market become (e.g. processed foods, white goods), the more important their cultural features become as a basis for choice between them. Recent marketing fashion has emphasized design, with products increasingly promoted in terms of both functional and cultural characteristics. One recent advertisement asks what car does the man who designs cars drive to work in from his home in a converted monastery? A single image associates the car with both design excellence and social status. To specify the functional and the cultural characteristics of a product is to specify how far the product will meet its user's needs: and this is to specify product quality.[45]

Promotion

Promotion is the second of McCarthy's four marketing tools and often the costliest: in US airlines up to 14% of revenue,[46] in UK pharmaceuticals up to 20%.[47] Changing British Airway's corporate livery alone cost in the range £25–£30 million.[48] In a commercial setting the heart of promotion is selling techniques, among which branding, merchandising and packaging are standard. Packaging is also designed both functionally (to protect and dispense the product) and culturally, to reinforce the image of the product as meeting the functional, emotional, social and other needs of the buyer. Branding attempts to get the user to associate a generic product (say vacuum cleaners) with a particular supplier's product (e.g. Hoover's).

Merchandising consists in so presenting the product as to maximize sales. Partly this is done at the point of sale. Many supermarkets place the most profitable lines at eye level and at the ends of aisles or place every day items far away from the entrance and contrive the shopper's route to them to pass displays of items known to attract impulse buying.[49]

Primarily the task of promotion is to recommend the product to potential buyers. A standard advertising method is to associate the product with a cultural as well as a functional benefit. Soap, for instance, is tacitly advertised as offering beauty or hope besides cleanliness.[50] Financial, industrial relations or political reasons also lead promotion to be often directed at secondary audiences such as shareholders (e.g. the recent privatizations), workforces, the government or the political public and the media. Paid advertisements and public relations methods can be used for both types of audience.

Public relations methods include using news conferences or 'events' to attract free editorial coverage, obtaining free editorial coverage in exchange for a certain quantity of advertising or backing pressure groups whose interests coincide with the firm's (e.g. some tobacco firms have sponsored FOREST, which advocates freedom of choice for smokers[51]). Until recently for instance, Marks and Spencer, used its public relations work almost exclusively for promoting its corporate image as a respectable, established firm responsible to the local community.

Price

Price can also be used as a promotional tool. Consumers sometimes imagine (often wrongly) that a higher priced item is of higher quality. Thus some products (e.g. perfume) can even increase their sales when prices are raised. Against this, the reader will be familiar with firms offering reductions in price to sustain sales during lulls in the business cycle or to clear a nearly obsolete product. In some markets, price is itself an important symbol (of social status). The 'executive' car market provides examples.

However, price is a major marketing tool (and third of McCarthy's four) in its own right. Price is one criterion by which markets can be segmented, and hence one important criterion by which products are designed. This applies not only at the functional level (e.g. because only a certain degree of accuracy in a camera lens is attainable for a given price) but also at the cultural level. Some products have been designed to look more expensive than they really are, as in the mass production of fake labels during the fashion for 'designer' clothing, or to make a virtue out of cheapness (e.g. the fashion for 'simple' food packaging in the 1970s). Pricing has other uses too. British Gas charges nothing for the first half hour of repair worker's time so as not to discourage requests for safety work. The way in which price is charged can also increase sales. Consumer credit not only makes it possible to sell sooner to the customer who lacks ready cash but also reduces the anxiety and sense of finality about large purchases by seeming to break the cost up into less alarming portions.[52]

Place

Place is the remaining marketing tool. In marketing the term has three main senses. The oldest and core sense concerns methods of distributing the product. Producers of fast moving consumer goods have to decide, for instance, whether to sell through major department stores, through franchising, through general retail outlets, direct mail order or whatever. Because services are neither transportable nor storable distribution questions in service industries resolve mainly into questions of where to situate work places and how to maximize buyer access (e.g. by the provision of car parking, creche, or information that the service is available and where).

A second aspect of place is the time at which the marketing strategy is to be implemented. Lead time for developing new products, and the lead or lag which competitors have from doing this is one time constraint; how long it takes for the market to respond to a new marketing strategy another. This constraint obviously depends upon the type of product, the time-scale over which it is consumed (days for food, years for cars) and the reasons for which consumers buy it. Marketing strategies, especially promotional strategies, also wear out. The impact of, say, a television advertisement increases up to a point with repetition but then falls away as viewers become desensitized.

'Place' can lastly refer to 'positioning' within a market. This refers to the development of certain product characteristics which differentiate this producer's goods from its competitors'. For example a stereo equipment manufacturer might seek a distinctive profile in terms of the set of characteristics by which stereo buyers judge stereos. It might position its product at one end of each of the continua 'cheap' *versus* 'expensive', 'basic' *versus* 'high specification' and 'popular' *versus* 'enthusiast' product. Once again market research can be used to establish what market position a firm's goods actually have, and what market positioning is likely to give the firm greatest competitive advantage.

A marketing strategy consisting of these tools has four noteworthy characteristics. Firstly the strategy is shaped by empirical market research which in turn is shaped by the organization's objectives, and shapes day-to-day operations. Secondly the marketing strategy governs not only the obviously marketing matters (e.g. product styling, advertising) but the technical specification of the product or service and the firm's research and development programme. Because a commercial producer must also have an eye to competitors, a marketing strategy is (thirdly) fluid and subject to frequent review. Multidimensionality is the fourth characteristic. A marketing strategy contains elements both to respond to demand (e.g. product design) and attempt to influence it (promotion, including social marketing), making the notion of 'consumer sovereignty' rather a half-truth.

The next task is to consider the process by which commercial organizations tend to implement their marketing strategies.

Implementing the marketing plan

Selling

Having decided a product mix, the product has to be made then sold. Of these two processes selling is the distinctively marketing-related, and distinctively commercial, task. Five essential elements for implementing a marketing plan are: distribution of the product (or providing access to a service); advertising and public relations; rewarding marketing success; ensuring line management is marketing driven; and tracking.

Selling revolves around the arrangements for distributing the product. Which are the most effective distribution channels (e.g. selling through brokers, supermarkets, wholesalers, mail order or whatever) are decided on the basis of market research into customers' characteristics and buyer habits. A luxury food manufacturer whose main customers are middle-aged professionals might decide to concentrate distribution on those outlets which market research reveals these people use (e.g. out-of-town branches of Marks and Spencer, hotels and restaurants).

When a distributor or retailer stands between producer and customer, the firm has to decide on the balance between 'pull' and 'push' strategies in selling. A push strategy consists in getting the middle man to buy the product and leaving it to the retailer and distributor to sell to the final buyer. A pull strategy aims to attract the final buyer to seek the product from the middle man.

For a 'push' strategy and for selling direct to the end buyer a trained salesforce is necessary. Their training lies in two areas. One is knowledge of the product or service sold, its uses, its merits compared with competing products, the likely buyers, their demands and objections. The second area is knowledge of selling, including practical skills at each major part of the selling process: prospecting for possible customers; approaching them; presenting the product or service to them; handling customer objections; closing the sale and providing any follow-up service (e.g. handling queries or complaints).[53] Knowledge of this process comes from consumer and marketing research.

Advertisements are so familiar an adjunct to this that a brief mention will suffice, noting that advertising can also be had through subtle methods such as arranging for the product to be seen being used by characters in a television soap opera or sponsorship. Adverts address both the functional and the cultural attributes of the product, and do so both explicitly and subliminally.

Vignette 1.4   The commandments of Marks and Spencer

Marks and Spencer is a long established and respectable company, cautious and careful in its approach to new ideas for management methods and products. The norms which its staff are expected to adopt have evolved gradually. They are now summarized in eight 'commandments' which serve much the same publicity purposes, in addressing staff and public, as is served by other firms' 'mission statements' or 'philosophies'. Marks and Spencer's staff programmes reinforce the norms and the reasons for them, focusing on product knowledge, merchandising, politeness and inter-personal skills. It takes place weekly and is ongoing for all staff. The Marks and Spencer 'commandments' are:

- To provide a high standard of quality and value
- Display merchandise attractively and make shopping pleasant and easy for customers
- Provide *friendly* service from *well-trained, knowledgeable* and *efficient* staff
- Foster good human relations with customers, staff, suppliers and communities in which stores are situated
- Encourage suppliers to use the most modern and efficient production techniques and to develop a long-term relationship
- Support British Industry
- Provide staff with good conditions of employment and ensure they share in company success
- Seek to improve quality standards in all areas

Marks and Spencer's staff programmes reinforce the norms and the reasons for them, focusing on product knowledge, merchandising, politeness and inter-personal skills. It takes place weekly and is ongoing for all staff.

An advert showing (say) a brand of coffee being used by the wealthy and fashionable associates use of that brand with being wealthy and fashionable (although no such claim is actually stated), tempting the viewer to conclude that by buying this coffee he or she too can become more like the wealthy or fashionable person shown in the advert.

Marketers recommend that an advert should attract attention, interest the potential customer in the product, arouse his or her desire for the product and stimulate action (i.e. buying) to get it. Commercial advertisers therefore seek to get their adverts noticed, remembered and the product recognized both from the advert and (later) when offered for sale. A body of marketing research into communication, perception and semiotics underlies these techniques.

Public relations is directed primarily at secondary publics (e.g. during water privatization) but can also indirectly encourage product sales. The recent British Gas advertising campaign appears to have been intended to establish BG in the target audiences' minds during the interval after gas but before (competing) electricity producer privatization.

The same media can sometimes be used for public relations as for product adverts. Television adverts can serve either to promote a corporate image (e.g. ICI presenting itself as an innovator by global standards) or to further social marketing of commercial value to the sponsor (e.g. the Tobacco Advisory Council adverts on air pollution). Logos and other visual materials are designed to convey subliminal messages about the organization. For instance the different-coloured, new type face 'h' in the new BHS logo was apparently intended to suggest style, flair and modernity. 'Mission' statements (or more pretentiously, 'philosophy' statements) can be used as public relations tools as well as for communication to staff. Vignette 1.4 gives an example.

Internal communications run in parallel. As a figurehead the senior manager is often involved in the launch of a new marketing strategy or plan, in the training programmes around it. The head of personal banking in one of the big four banks was at one time spending two or three days a week presenting 'road shows', writing for the house magazine, and talking to and observing how front-line staff implemented its marketing plan in practice. In many commercial settings training concerns not only the development of skills but also an explanation of the firm's current marketing plan, why it is important and the benefits to be expected. Because line managers and staff implement the marketing plan, some organizations use them rather than personnel or marketing trainers to communicate the marketing plan through training channels. British Airways for example uses cabin crew and ground staff to explain their contribution to airline's work (see Vignette 1.5).

Motivation and management

Communications to staff provide psychological rewards for successful implementation of the marketing plan (or with bad management, the opposite).

Firms therefore report successes in their company newsletters and other internal media both as a motivator and as a positive model to staff. Other non-cash rewards include recognition and status of staff who contribute to implementing the marketing plan, so for example, performance stars and badges are conspicuous on McDonalds counter staff. All this represents the application for marketing purposes of general theories of motivation which the reader can also find in the many texts on the subject.[54]

Vignette 1.5   British Airways – The uses of training

The air travel market is highly competitive. Passengers' choices of airline depend largely on their experience of it and their expectations. The latter come partly from the potential customer's own perception of the airline and partly from recommendations of passengers who have in turn experienced travel with the airline recently. Anticipating privatization, British Airways concluded that it was necessary to re-examine the quality of its product, the quality of the environment for passengers and staff and the quality of the service. Improvements in the first two areas would, BA feared, be relatively easily copied by competitors and would not therefore give BA any lasting advantage. Higher quality of service would admittedly be harder to attain, but would give a competitive advantage that could be maintained with continued effort. Raising the quality of product and environment were also attempted but service quality was chosen for the flagship of BA's reform and publicity.

There was a thorough review of the airline's objectives, management structure and training. A Market Product Group was formed to focus on ideas for change. The Market Product Group was inter-occupational and thus able to suggest innovation in all the airline's activities. Groups of staff were formed charged with focussing on aspects of quality and the development of training programmes for staff. Among the service quality problems identified were hygiene and cleanliness on aeroplanes, punctuality and aircraft servicing. British Airways also wished to make its staff aware of the costs of each element in its operations a view to increasing financial control and profitability.

Market research was initiated to discover what the customers' view of British Airways was, what the airline staff's view of their customers expectations was, how BA staff perceived their own behaviour towards customers and how BA compared with its competitors on these points. It was found that staff views of what customers expected in terms of service, and what the customers actually expected differed considerably. It also showed a necessity to improve staff self-perception and strengthen their confidence in their ability to influence levels of customer satisfaction.

From these results were derived minimum services standards based on customers' own expectations. A staff training programme was also initiated among the staff who remained after the loss, in 1981–1982, of some 22 000 jobs (40% of the workforce). The programme was undertaken on a mass scale. Session presentations were largely by operational staff rather than trainers. Their purpose was to show staff in each part of the airline what staff in the other parts do, to give awareness of the approach to customer care required, and what staff can contribute.

Cash is a more obvious reward for marketing success. For salesmen and saleswomen it is common to make salaries a mixture of fixed rate and performance-related bonus. Some firms add occasional extras to this. One manufacturer for instance is known to offer successful salesmen and their families weekends at a hotel of their choice paid for by the firm.

For a marketing strategy to be implemented line managers must know how to base their daily decisions on marketing considerations and market research data (implying that the chief executive must understand marketing). It is therefore for the senior line managers to initiate and commission major pieces of market research. The results, including tracking results, have to be fed back to those who can initiate action upon them. This implies feedback to two main groups. Senior managers require the market research results to analyse how successfully the marketing plan is being implemented, to decide rewards, and to alter the production or distribution of the product, product design, advertising, public relations and the other marketing variables. Operational managers, sometimes down to supervisor level, require tracking feedback for making day to day service adjustments (e.g. redeployment of supermarket staff from shelf filling to the checkouts).

All the above activities require a supporting information system. Many

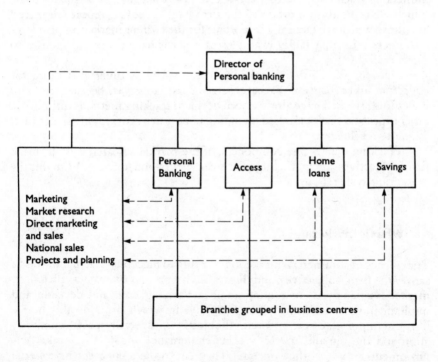

Figure 1.2 Part of the management structure of a major UK bank 1987

firms therefore have a marketing section at national or regional level responsible for tracking studies, marketing audit and drafting the marketing strategy and plan.

Figure 1.2 illustrates one firm's approach to these organizational matters. The central marketing function provides information to the director to enable him to monitor service provision overall and decide his subordinates' rewards. His subordinate managers have routine access to the information held by the marketing function that relates to their own customer segment.

Tracking

Tracking is a major activity of the central market researchers. If organized at regional or national level the collection and interpretation of tracking data is independent of those whose performance is tracked. Because the marketing objectives are multiple so are the monitoring indicators which are derived from these and so therefore are the data used to monitor or 'track' achievement of the marketing plan. However, it is rare for every aspect of the marketing plan to be tracked continuously. Often a manageably small number of tracking indicators are selected for each segment, usually those which are centrally important to the firm (e.g. turnover, repeat sales, etc.) and those which are tactically important for the current marketing plan (e.g. customers returning faulty examples of a particular product, responses to direct mail).

Methods for collecting tracking data can be as diverse as those for collecting other forms of market research data. However, because the main issues to be tracked have already been decided, tracking methods differ from other types of research method intending to be much more highly structured. Vignette 1.6 illustrates this.

Tracking data is one component of the market research by which the firm's objectives and marketing plan are reviewed and updated. With this the marketing cycle repeats.

What is marketing?

The essence of commercial marketing is trying to meet buyer demand so as to satisfy the firm's objectives; and this through a process of business planning, market-type analysis, marketing audit and strategizing, and devising and implementing a marketing plan. The ways in which firms do this bear a heavy stamp both of their structural objectives (especially profit maximization and the pursuit of effective buyer demand) and of the market environments in which they operate. They constitute a coherent managerial process by which the firm meets these objectives by manipulating the market relation between the goods or services it produces and the user of these goods and services to achieve a match between the two.

Vignette 1.6   Tracking Tesco

Tesco launched its 'Checkout' campaign in 1977 and after first raising its market share from 7% to 14% then falling back to slightly above 11%, Tesco concluded that it could gain no further market share by holding down prices and indeed its market share would remain vulnerable if it depended on price setting alone. Increased business would therefore depend on non-price aspects of customer service and quality.

For some years Tesco have participated in joint market research with other retail organizations. Carried out quarterly, this research concentrated on customer image and service. In the late 1970s Tesco consistently came among the also-rans with ratings some 15% below those of Safeway, Sainsburys and Waitrose. Tesco recognized that if they were to displace Sainsbury as the top UK supermarket group they would have to shift customer perceptions that Tesco offered low prices at the expense of quality of products and of service. A new customer-service strategy resulted, combining a high-profile launch in 1987 with emphasis on subsequent consolidation.

Monitoring is evidently the key to consolidating the customer service strategy. Tesco has adopted an extensive 'ghost shopper' approach. Head office staff armed with a checklist each visit a designated number of stores annually. The materials used for monitoring (and for internal communications) are of a high quality, detailed and specific. For instance there is a checklist for monitoring whether staff adopt the specified procedure for handling a customer complaint. The main actions monitored are; acknowledgement (verbally and non-verbally), action taken, staff appearance and whether the outcome is satisfactory. Similar lists are used to monitor the behaviours of counter staff, how staff deal with customer requests for a product or for information, checking-out and the physical environment.

Data collected by the ghost shoppers are recorded in the central computer. Detailed results are copied to the relevant store and headquarters managers. Summaries are published in the staff magazine. All this is supplemented with continuing image perception research besides the usual indicators of cash flow, sales volume and market share.

Yet this process is carried out in many different ways depending on such diverse factors as the nature of the product, the history and circumstances of the firm and the type of markets and environments in which the firm operates. Each firm therefore selects from the repertoire of marketing knowledge and techniques those suited to its present strategy. Not all of these selections and techniques are relevant to publicly funded health services.

The common factor to the different applications of marketing in the commercial sector is as a managerial process. In this process the organization's objectives determine how markets are analysed through market research, how and why marketing audit is undertaken and how and why the marketing plan and its implementation (plan and implementation comprising what we have called the 'techniques' of marketing) are put into effect. This process is almost always iterative with a feedback cycle through market

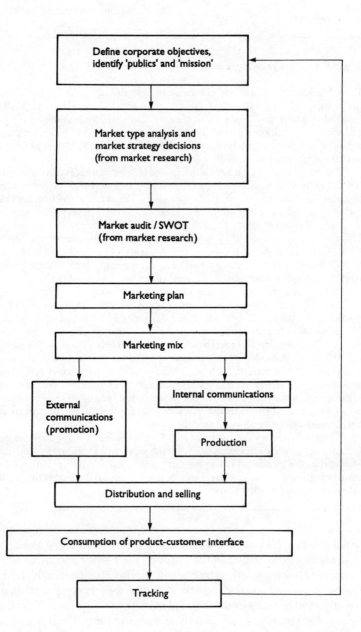

Figure 1.3 Marketing – the commercial prototype

research and tracking. The whole process is flexible in the sense of encouraging the adaptation of new techniques both in production and in marketing in the light of technical and market changes. The background body of marketing research, besides competitor's experience and firm's own inventiveness provide the repertoire from which these adaptations are drawn. Figure 1.3 gives a simplified illustration of this process.

Figure 1.3 outlines the generic model of marketing at the integrative level. The branch in this cycle should not be interpreted as an 'either-or' decision between using internal or external communications. Both will be required in most applications, although with a different balance of emphasis according to circumstances. Insofar as the marketing strategy requires an attempt to stimulate demand or change its character, it will have to emphasize external communication. Insofar as marketing strategy emphasizes altering the goods and services produced to meet existing demands, internal communications and reward systems will require emphasis. This is just one respect in which the model in Figure 1.3 is a formal model of a high level or generality, capable of accepting different interpretations in, and being adapted to, very different circumstances.

By 'marketing' most NHS staff – like most of the general public – would probably understand something like 'advertising' or 'salesmanship', as the above account of commercial marketing would seem to confirm, although these aspects are only the public face of commercial marketing. Even one of the narrowest standard definitions takes 'marketing' as 'the performance of business activities that direct the flow of goods from the producer to consumer or user',[55] a definition already wider than the range of NHS innovations listed on pp. 1–5. To use 'marketing' as a short generic label for them demands a provisional definition of marketing broad enough to include non-commercial, non-profit organizations, pending further investigation of what precisely the word means.

Philip Kotler, arguably the leading US writer on health care marketing, provides a possible definition:

> *Marketing* is the analysis, planning, implementation and control of carefully formulating programs designed to bring about voluntary exchanges of values with target markets for the purpose of achieving organizational objectives. It relies heavily on designing the organization's offering in terms of the target markets' needs and desires, and on using effective pricing, communication and distribution to inform, motivate and service the markets.[56]

By 'market' Kotler appears to mean any social domain within which 'voluntary exchanges of values' are sought, not only markets in the narrower, everyday sense of the word; and that these exchanges are not limited to monetary exchanges. Elsewhere he defines 'values' too in non-monetary terms.[57] Kotler's definition, however, conflates of 'need' with 'wishes' and both with 'effective demand'. This obscures a fundamental set of distinctions for the NHS and for internal markets. Instead of using Kotler's faintly justificatory terms 'inform' and 'service' it would be as well to leave it open whether commercial and NHS marketing is to the user's advantage or disadvantage. Kotler's jargon of 'exchange', 'markets' and 'value' suggests a link with social interactionist theory with which NHS marketing does not have to be lumbered.

For the NHS and organizations like it a more applicable and coherent definition of 'marketing' is:

> Marketing: the managerial cycle whereby an organization attempts to meet its objectives by so designing its products and so influencing potential takers of its product that the product and relevant taker characteristics match.

'Organization' covers commercial, statutory and voluntary organizations. 'Product' should be taken to include services or social objectives besides physical products. 'Takers' can be buyers, the actual product user, or the targets of promotional campaigns. Their 'relevant characteristics' may be psychological, behavioural or social. Above all the proposed definition implies that to recommend marketing to the NHS is not to recommend market provision of health care; it may do the opposite.

There remains the problem of whether to use commercial marketing jargon in NHS contexts. The lesser evil, given NHS interest in parallels with commercial marketing, is to follow NHS managers and retain this jargon in NHS use. But as NHS marketing develops there will be much to be said for devising a jargon less ambiguous and less open to political abuse.

Defining 'marketing' is not for present purposes a merely verbal, theoretical matter[58] because it reflects a major practical question. This is, whether the activities which in a commercial organization would conventionally be called 'marketing' need to be carried out so differently in a non-commercial (non-profit) health service that the term 'marketing' would be misleading. This presumes that marketing can and should be attempted in the NHS at all. To understand how marketing can be practised in the NHS these questions must first be confronted.

Chapter 2

Can marketing apply to NHS health care? And should it?

Objections to marketing NHS health care

Health care as a special good

Some objections to marketing NHS health care commonly arise. They either arise from considering health care an atypical good or find marketing inherently objectionable, or arise from the institutional peculiarities of the NHS.

Economic objections hold that health care cannot be efficiently distributed by markets nor, therefore, by methods involving marketing, for marketing is essentially an ancillary to commerce.[1] (Some writers actually define marketing as a commercial activity (see chapter 1, p. 29). Not only do markets allocate health care resources inefficiently but marketing exaggerates the maldistribution because market research is largely pseudoscientific.[2] Consumers are ignorant about diagnosis, treatment, asymptomatic disease, the quality of care[3] and doctors' skill.[4] Major treatments tend to be once-off events[5] providing little opportunity for the patients to learn from experience[6] except in palpable failure of care.[7] Many patients anyway refuse to 'own' serious illness and prefer to abdicate responsibility for decisions to a professional.[8] Consumers cannot always know or anticipate their demand for health care so price decisions cannot work as economic theory supposes.[9] Consumers may have a right to care, or be compelled to receive it.[10] Consumer decisions made in such conditions are likely to maximize neither the user's welfare nor economic efficiency.

In commercial health systems, consumer ignorance and patients' often deferential attitudes to doctors[11] leaves sellers of health care unusual scope to defraud the consumer. Promotion and sales techniques reinforce consumer irrationality for instance by appealing to 'hidden needs' for (say) reassurance or social status, 'impulse selling' or spuriously associating the product with irrelevant effects such as enhanced sexual attractiveness.[12] Aneurin Bevan remarked that he would prefer to survive in a large impersonal hospital than expire amid a gush of sympathy in a small one and a similar objection can be made to well marketed but clinically inappropriate health services.[13] A common selling ploy is to arouse the consumer's anxiety so that the provider can then claim to offer a product that relieves it.[14] BUPA have come under Advertising Standards Authority scrutiny for hinting at NHS inadequacies for such purposes.[15] Health care is most obviously demanded when a person is ill but illness often reduces the consumer's capacity for informed and rational decision (see above). Consumers are least likely to exercise choice when they are actually in contact with health services for fear of antagonizing the doctor when he or she is most needed.[16]

Some marketers promote ill health. Peter Taylor quotes a US market research firm's advice to the makers of 'Viceroy' cigarettes:

> Full flavour smokers perceive smoking as dangerous to their health . . .
> Given their awareness of the smoking and health situation, they are faced with the fact that they are acting illogically. . . .
>
> *Advertising Objective* To Communicate effectively that VICEROY is a satisfying, flavourful cigarette which young adult smokers enjoy, by providing them a rationalization for smoking, or, a repression of the health concern they appear to need.[17]

Other economic objections concern commercial health care only. Interpersonal comparisons affect the utility arising from health-care decisions. Doctors act both as supplier of the service and as interpreter and representative of the patient's needs. Here supply and demand are not independent. Then markets do not work in (what most economists regard as) the normal, utility-maximizing ways.[18] When ill health incapacitates, the individual's demand for health care is greatest when there is least capacity to pay.

Ethical objections

One consumer remedy for ignorance and irrationality is to delegate their health care decisions to professionals.[19] The objection that marketing activities conflict with professional considerations would make marketing unimplementable in health care.[20] The BMA ethical code still forbids doctors' adverts to imply that one doctor has better skills or knowledge than another, forbids promoting commercial organizations in which the doctor has an interest or sharing buildings with commercial organizations and curtails advertising generally.[21] Professional ethics suppose that the patient's trust is necessary to a proper relationship between professional and patient, and salesmanship which would reduce it to the levels attributed to advertising executives and estate agents.[22]

Marketing techniques are designed to increase demand for services, especially those with maximum value added but since nearly all health care is iatrogenic NHS marketing is undesirable.[23] The doctrine of clinical autonomy arose partly to protect doctors and patients from extraneous, commercial influences on clinical decisions and standards of care, to enable clinicians to decide a treatment or care plan solely with regard to the interests of the individual patient in front of him or her.[24] To show that marketing NHS services would prejudice clinical autonomy would be a most damaging objection because it would imply that health-care marketing defeats its own rationale of safeguarding and improving patient care. It is often alleged that marketing considerations on behalf of private care do prejudice clinical autonomy in the NHS,[25] that patients are let believe that even clinically necessary treatment will be had sooner by 'going private'. Anxiety has been expressed that both the clumsier forms of clinical audit and the increased managerial concern for quality would also compromise clinical autonomy and patient care.[26]

There are wider ethical objections to marketing health care. Norman Daniels assumes that a market system can function as welfare economics intends only if all participants have equal opportunity. This requires the provision of the medical care necessary to maintain humans' normal 'species' function.[27] (This implies a wider definition of health care than as medical care of sickness only.[28]) So health care should be provided according to a principle of equal opportunity,[29] removing market obstacles to initial access to health care.[30]

Richard Titmuss[31] argued that the system of donating blood as a gift without coercion or constraint and out of motives of social solidarity yields blood of a higher quality without coercion or constraint.[32] A market in blood

> represses the expression of altruism, erodes the sense of community, lowers scientific standards, limits both personal and professional freedoms, sanctions the making of profits in hospitals and clinical laboratories, legalizes hostility between doctor and patient, subjects critical areas of medicine to the laws of the marketplace, places immense social costs on those least able to bear them . . . increases the danger of unethical behaviour in various sectors of medical science and practice[33]

This raises the question of whether using marketing methods more widely in the NHS would also reproduce these effects throughout it.

Objections to marketing

These objections hold that commercial marketing uses largely disreputable methods of which consumer deception is only the crudest. This can take the form of straightforward untruthfulness. In 1971 the US Food and Drug Administration found no evidence for the therapeutic claims made for 60% of the products it examined.[34] UK manufacturers mislabel the active ingredient in anti-smoking aids as 'purified tobacco' not 'nicotine'[35] and so on. There is more than a hint of trickery in 'bait and switch' and subliminal selling.[36] Kotler and Clarke say that 'marketers recognise that consumers cannot be sold something they don't need or want';[37] critics doubt it. Many adverts convey only illogical and non-factual messages; 'The game is to be promising something you aren't without actually lying.'[38], for instance by using a comparative without stating its comparitor or using the 'hedge word', by juxtaposing two imperatives to suggest a (spurious) connection (e.g. 'Chip-pendale in the study, Strachan in the bedroom'[39]) or asking a leading rhetorical question (e.g. 'Can you face another boring lunchtime snack?'[40]) Anticipating the effects of health-care advertising in the USA the Council of Medical Specialty Services issued guidelines which classify as fraudulent those adverts which omit material facts, exaggerate the degree of recovery attainable by the average patient or the very possibility of cure, falsely suggest that a physician's qualification or skill is above average, those which conceal the fact that they are paid adverts and those which understate or partly conceal patient fees payable.[41]

Marketers are accused of designing for 'acceptability' to the lowest common denominators of taste (so reinforcing them),[42] of devaluing and evacuating language (the London Underground no longer displays 'maps' but 'journey planners'). Advertisers target on children to 'club' parents into buying.[43] Feminists object that by associating the product for sale with a supposedly positive symbol (e.g. an 'attractive' young woman) the advert also suggests that the associated symbol is to be interpreted positively, so reinforcing sexist stereotypes of women. Most product redesigns are trivial, intended mainly to make previous models 'psychologically obsolete'.[44] 'Planned obsolescence', adulteration and the sacrifice of safety standards are used to make goods more saleable. Packard argued that when the American car industry adopted marketing on a large-scale in the 1950s every aspect of car quality deteriorated except engine characteristics, and these were deter-mined by technicians not marketers.[45] Kotler and Clarke defend health-care marketing by tacitly redefining 'marketing' as 'sales promotion' and then arguing that not only poor products get promoted.[46] This misses the objection's point. 'Consumerist' groups emerged in the 1960s not to promote marketing but to protect consumers from it. A consumerist NHS would not embrace marketing but resist it.[47]

There remain some contingent objections. Modern NHS experience in generating income and donations suggests that the easiest services to market to sources of income outside NHS (insurers, employers, public appeals), and the easiest to market politically, are those such as maternity and children's services, transplants and high-technology curative medicine generally which have an easily intelligible appeal for the public, and then in the wealthier localities. Such marketing techniques and experience as the NHS has are further developed there, more familiar and likelier to be applied successfully by NHS managers. Marketing for income generation outside the 'internal' market will tend to recreate the maldistributions caused by market failure up to 1938 and since the middle 1970s. These tendencies are likely to be strengthened by the coming of the internal market and the concomitant marketing activity, especially if NHS service providers have to compete with existing commercial providers on their terms. To start marketing NHS services is to step onto a slippery slope that ends in a market health system. Besides, governments are likelier to use marketing of NHS services as a cosmetic for existing health policy rather than to assist the NHS in meeting consumer demands and needs, as the launch publicity and presentation media for *Working For Patients* itself, for the Resource Management Initiative and for other health policies indicates.

An opposite objection takes the NHS as a special, non-commercial case to which marketing will remain largely irrelevant even after *Working for Patients* is implemented. Even in the 'internal' market conventional marketing seems inapplicable because the 'service contracts' will have to be a largely cosmetic addition to the existing planning system, and marketing will remain totally irrelevant to the user–provider interface.[48] Yet it is from its effects at this interface that marketing derives its main justification (of satisfying consumer demands). The NHS remains virtually a monopoly for many types of service and even after the implementation of *Working for Patients* is likely to remain so for the uninsured majority, for the uninsurable and for those who refuse private health care – some 85% of the UK population on 1988 figures.[49]

Either way, the objection arises that when demand for care exceeds NHS resources, marketing wastes resources that could be put to clinical use. Suppose the NHS adopted marketing on a scale at the lower end of the range of percentages of income that commercial organizations devote to marketing by allocating 2% of its income to marketing activities. On 1986–1987 figures this is equivalent to the mean cost of treating approximately 597 000 inpatients at a time when waiting lists exceeded 680 000.[50] NHS services are already overloaded without attracting more 'customers' through marketing, even admitting exceptions such as marketing to increase uptake blood and organ donation, health promotion or vaccination and immunization programmes. Even if one did wish to attract more work to NHS hospitals, increasing the provision of NHS care alone seems to achieve this; for all the rises and falls in beddage the length of NHS waiting lists has remained more or less stable since 1947.[51]

Finally the NHS is already doing well in satisfying the public as opinion polls show consistently over more than two decades.[52] Compared with alternative health systems the successes of the NHS in meeting consumer demands and needs are evident enough.

After all these subtractions of elements of marketing that cannot or should not be applied in the NHS, it might be concluded, not much remains: certainly too little to make it worthwhile installing marketing as a major function of NHS management. How valid is this formidable catalogue of objections to marketing in the NHS?

The objections assessed

The condition of the NHS

Some objections are easily demolished. That the NHS is a monopoly and popular is no objection to trying to improve upon its successes, even by marketing methods, especially since scope for improvement remains.

Vignette 2.1   A visit to the accident and emergency department

A late middle-aged gentlemen injured himself at home one Saturday evening
and made his way to the accident and emergency department at the town's main
acute hospital. The receptionist, who was courteous and considerate, asked him
to sit down and wait until his name was called. He found the waiting area rather
small and shabby, and none too clean. The only things to read whilst he waited
were in Asian languages – of little use to someone whose only language is
English. Apart from a number of drunken youths swearing and occasionally
fighting no other diversion was available during the long wait. Mr A had lived
in the town all his life and used the accident emergency services some 30 years
before. The waiting time was just as long then. However there was a telephone
and after waiting 15 minutes for someone else to finish with it Mr A was able to
use it. The phone box door was spring loaded. It opened easily enough but
closed suddenly, striking him in the back. The telephone itself was by then out
of order.

Eventually Mr A was seen. One of the nurses he met had rather a matronly
manner. Another, apparently a young trainee, seemed to him rather apathetic.
Nevertheless most of the clinical staff seemed efficient and helpful. The doctor
ordered an X-ray. The woman in the X-ray room seemed 'a little sharp' but
once the X-ray was done the doctor gave him all the information he wanted
about the injury and his condition. The local anaesthetic seemed rather ineffective – almost as painful as the injury itself. But for Mr A the most important
thing was that his injury was eventually cured. He had expected first-class
medical treatment and was satisfied that he had received it. Altogether Mr A
spent several hours in the department.

These events took place in a university town in the Midlands in July 1988.

(Vignettes 2.1 and 2.2 illustrate some of the areas.) Performance indicators,
such NHS market research data as are available and administrative data
indicate that difficulties of the kind illustrated there are far from rare.

It might be replied that they have less to do with marketing than with
shortage of cash. Real resources available for the NHS have fallen since 1980
allowing for demographic shifts, technological changes and the relative price
effect,[53] but how much extra NHS funding is necessary to resolve the
problem cannot be answered without a knowledge of user needs and
demands and the service changes necessary to meet them. Market research,
and marketing theory, are needed for this and to diagnose the problems
which the shortages putatively create.

Besides, such difficulties with NHS services still occurred when the
NHS had an open-ended access to cash on a call-off basis as a reading of many
official reports from before 1976 will confirm.[54] So these problems arise not
simply from cash shortage but have organizational roots. No organizational
method for meeting user demands and needs systematically has ever been
structured into the NHS. Its founders apparently assumed that clinicians
would act as patient advocates. That may be plausible in regard to clinical care
but less so in regard to the non-clinical aspects. CHCs, Health Authorities

and Parliamentary control are instruments too crude to achieve the complex and subtle service changes required. The remedy must be one which integrates and organizes existing management activity around the definition of user needs and demands, the implementation of action to meet these needs and demands, monitoring the results and doing all this routinely and centrally. Marketing appears to offer a solution.

Government are increasingly marketing their health policies whether the NHS does or not. The only question is whether the NHS replies in kind, developing these methods for its own uses and as a corrective to government claims when necessary. The NHS and health professionals already see no objection in principle to using their high public standing when generating income or (in the case of the BMA) lobbying to oppose *Working for Patients*.

What NHS marketing cannot achieve

Marketing should not be over-sold to the NHS, nor rejected for failing to achieve purposes for which it was never intended. For example, social marketing can only influence the funding of NHS services indirectly. Marketing cannot obviate trade offs between the cost, quantity, quality and mixture of different care options, but only provide a managerial process which places user demands and needs higher in these decisions. Neither can

---

Vignette 2.2   Elsie's experience

As part of its initiatives to 'personalize' NHS services in the Region, Trent RHA commissioned the Line-up communications consultancy to produce an awareness raising and training media package. The handbook shows staff and patients at Doncaster Royal Infirmary re-enacting the hospital experiences of Elsie, an elderly surgical patient. Elsie is shown having a long wait for her hospital treatment, and then a long wait in a slightly run-down clinic before two hurried and rather uninformative consultations with doctors. A year later and after one false alarm about being called in for her operation, Elsie is admitted to hospital (a rather disorganized process). After a postponement and a number of other more minor inconveniences, she is operated on and discharged home as chaotically as she was admitted.

Elsie is a fictional character but the results of such market research as is available elsewhere in the NHS suggests that Elsie's story is realistic. To make her list of misfortunes still more representative one might also mention the lack of privacy during consultations, the lack of reading material or other diversion during the long waits at out-patient clinics, the incivility of her GP's receptionist and the overbooking of both clinics and ambulances. However, there are also successes to, add: the care and attention given by staff is mentioned again and again by many respondents and, in many hospitals, the flexibility of waiting arrangements.

Sources: Trent Regional Health Authority *From Me to You* Sheffield 1987; NHS survey material at Health Services Management Unit, Manchester University.

marketing resolve the conflict of interest between management and staff over pay, conditions of employment, etc., which is not specific to the NHS, nor cheapen the provision of health care per unit of service of a given quality. (Creating a marketing function would initially increase these costs.) Neither is marketing a substitute for the recapitalization or re-equipment of under-funded services, nor for training and rewarding staff adequately.

Overload and under-resourcing of the NHS are valid objections to NHS marketing if, but only if, cost benefit analyses show that the cost of NHS marketing would *necessarily* outweigh any resulting saving due to increased service impact. Whether this is so is not obvious *a priori*.

Is marketing in the NHS a step onto a slippery slope towards privatiz-ation of the NHS? The assumptions that even if a commercialized health system is not intended it is likely to be the actual result of White Paper implementation, and that marketing is one component of this process, can all be accepted. This is an objection to marketing NHS services if, but only if, one already objects to White Paper implementation on other grounds. Marketing in the internal market between service buyer and provider will probably have to take a different form to marketing at the interface between service and non-paying user (see Chapter 3 and beyond). Applications of social marketing by the NHS could end in strengthening it against both political attrition and commercial competitors. Whether this happens depend upon exactly what forms of marketing the NHS eventually develops and what uses NHS managers put them to.

Marketing and commercial health care

The remaining objections are not easily gainsaid. They gain force from linking marketing with markets and hence with the least defensible aspects of private health care and commercial marketing. Insofar as the negative aspects of marketing stem from its commercial uses the only redress would be to find a way of separating marketing from commerce. So in principle market-ing might be a more effective way to meet consumer needs and demands outside markets than through them. If so, the NHS and similar organizations have a marketing advantage over commercial organizations. Because the NHS is only now beginning to apply marketing it has the opportunity to avoid or minimize the negative factors. Commercial marketing also has many gaps for NHS purposes. Its methods for analysing user needs, and needs for health care specifically, remain underdeveloped compared both with its methods for assessing effective demand and with the requirements of NHS planning.

The available practical experience and theoretical knowledge suggests that marketing is feasible in non-commercial, non-profit organizations. There are many examples in the US literature and practice alone, and Vignettes 1.4 and 6.1 give two British instances.[55] The NHS already applies some marketing practices unwittingly. Meeting user demands and needs already figures among the main objectives of the NHS and the ethos of patient care is strong. Clinical professionals already accept some marketing tasks: evaluating the outcome of health care, setting and raising standards for clinical care, considering user needs in producing operational policies and checking user experience of the resulting services, and social marketing to promote health behaviours and health policy.

The NHS requires a special form of marketing

Marketing can and should be applied to NHS services but simply imitating commercial marketing is unlikely to be successful or desirable. A hybrid form of marketing is required for the NHS and comparable organizations. (Besides its practical importance for health services the development of such a hybrid is also important for the status of the marketing discipline.) The reasons for marketing NHS services, the objections and replies outlined above suggest that NHS marketing would have to:

1 Make benefits to NHS users the central objective and rationale of NHS management, defining 'benefits' and hence service quality and marketing objectives in terms of user needs, by contrast with the commercial focus on effective demand (which many marketing writers confuse with needs[56]). The distinction between users' needs and their wishes is complex but following chapters take user wishes as an (occasionally unreliable) expression of user needs.[57]
2 Ensure the clinical neutrality of marketing methods, conserving clinical autonomy defined as the clinician's freedom to place individual patient needs above other criteria in deciding treatment plans.
3 Enable swift, practical responses to changes in user wishes and needs.
4 Enable alternative patterns of service to become available within the NHS, partly to provide continual innovation, partly as a means of reflecting the actual diversity in user needs and demands.
5 Enable the NHS to influence users' demands towards health services where this is likely to improve the users' health status through encouraging compliance or altering user knowledge or behaviour. Social marketing is required to advance health policy and intersectoral objectives through the political arena. Anti-marketing is a necessary part of health promotion; it will be unpopular with the marketing and advertising establishments but these are not strongly placed to complain about unethical methods.
6 Level up access to health care on the basis of need, for example by using segmentation and other marketing methods as a medium for positive discrimination.
7 Allow demarketing because of the overload of some NHS services but the onus of proof that this will not harm NHS users should be on those who propose to demarket a service.
8 Make 'interactive marketing', with its emphasis on staff development central to NHS marketing because personal care is the core 'technology' of health services.[58]

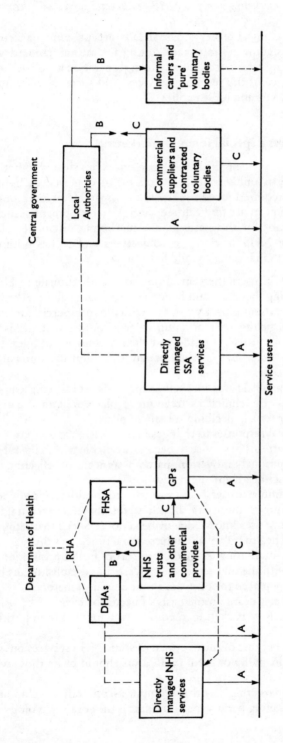

Figure 2.1 Types of marketing interface in the NHS internal market after 1991

9 Proscribe 'unethical' commercial marketing techniques (e.g. creating psychological obsolescence) and misleading advertising and promoting techniques; and to exploit only health-related motives in promotions and marketing, not encourage (e.g.) organ donation or service use for non-health motives.

Following chapters attempt to reinterpret the generic model of marketing (In Figure 1.3) along the above lines for NHS use in the 1990s. The resulting hybrid is intended to escape the objections discussed above and to be adapted to an NHS setting.

Three distinct but related variants of NHS marketing will be required after 1991: a buyer variant, a seller variant and a variant for directly-managed services. All three variants derive from the generic model in Figure 1.3. Common to all three are the activities of objective setting, market research, deriving operational policies, a promotional strategy and tracking (although these have to be done differently in each variant). Accounts of the buyer and

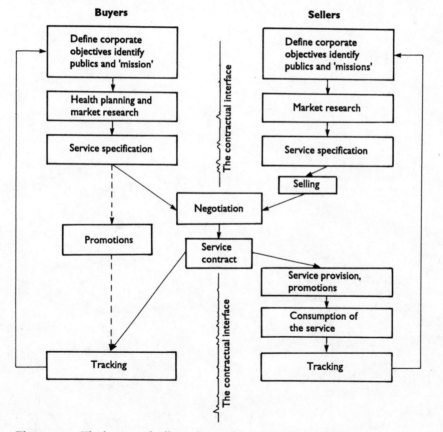

Figure 2.2 The buyer and seller variants of the NHS marketing model: a simplified overview

sellers necessarily has a more speculative tone until the implementation details for *Working for Patients*, particularly for hospital trusts, and specimen service contracts are finalized. Figure 2.1 illustrates the different parts of the NHS to which each variant would apply in the internal market.

The directly managed variant still applies to the great bulk of the NHS at the time of writing (early 1990), to directly managed local authority and voluntary body community care and to GPs in their capacity as providers of primary care. It is likely to make greater use of demarketing, social marketing and antimarketing methods than most commercial marketing does. The buyer and seller variants divide the steps in Figure 1.3 between them (but with some duplication) as Figure 2.2 shows. The seller variant applies not only to SGTs but to voluntary bodies; also to general practices that sell secondary care. The next four chapters explain the practicalities of the three variants in greater detail.

Chapter 3

Marketing NHS health care; objective setting through market research

Practical preliminaries

Initial decisions

The practical concerns of NHS marketers differ from those of commercial marketing. This chapter considers how to start addressing marketing and quality issues practically through service contracting in the internal market. It assumes that the NHS reader is attempting these activities for the first time and may decide to begin with a single department or service. To begin an NHS marketing project six initial decisions have to be taken:

Which service to begin with?

GPs have less scope for choice but in a hospital or community service the best choice is a discrete, self-contained service within which any difficulties are likely to be containable (e.g. A&E, physiotherapy). Since the first attempt may be regarded as a pilot it is obviously wise to select a service where success is likelier (e.g. where medical staff already support the idea of marketing) and whose problems and management structure are fairly representative. This does not preclude selecting the first area for intervention on a problem-solving basis (e.g. starting with OPD because of the level of complaints). If new expenditure has already been earmarked for a service (e.g. for a large capital scheme or staff training) this service may be a good starting point because resources are available to implement recommendations generated through market research.

Who to involve in marketing?

The line manager of the service, or the deputy, must accept responsibility for the marketing work at the level of the department or service. If a marketing or quality specialist is involved it should be as adviser or consultant to this manager.[1] The latter will need figurehead support from the UGM, DGM,

HA chairperson and from leading medical figureheads. No less important is to explain to staff at the outset what will happen, the reasons for embarking on marketing, who is going to be involved, what will happen, why and the possible outcomes. The purpose is to make intelligible to staff the contribution expected from them and the benefits to them and to patients.

What resources to allocate?

This obviously depends on the size of service selected but the requirements for a middle-sized OPD give a clue. To complete the marketing cycle outlined at the end of Chapter 2 one should allow about 30 days of management time plus whatever training the responsible manager needs. Administrative or secretarial support may be required for the production of questionnaires and other market research documents and for the other tasks outlined below. It may be possible to begin market research (i.e. step 5B in Figure 3.1) about three months from starting but consultations with clinicians and staff may double this. For market researching one department or service at unit level a budget in the range of £2000 to £5000 should be set aside for printing, postage, hospitality for volunteers, etc. plus the costs of outside consultancy if used. At the outset one must also resource any parallel evaluation of the marketing work and have contingency plans for resourcing whatever training or other service changes the market research indicates. Expect to pay over £3000 for an independent evaluation.

Will the marketing activity be evaluated independently?

Any marketing work whose decisions are made on the basis of market research, and which includes a tracking system, thereby generates its own internal method for evaluating the steps taken to act upon the market research findings. Additionally, and especially in a first-time project, it may also be desirable to have the whole process evaluated independently by an academic or a consultancy (e.g. to guide decisions whether or how to extend the marketing work). The decision on this *must* be taken at the outset otherwise evaluation using 'before' and 'after' data is impossible.

Are we capable of attempting marketing to a high standard?

At this stage many NHS managers doubt in their ability to undertake marketing and market research to a high standard. Yet even a fairly slow or inefficient attempt at marketing will be a large improvement over previous conditions (no marketing at all) and marketing skills can partly be developed through practice.

What preparatory training is required for the staff who will do marketing?

Training in marketing methods and management, may be required to elucidate what is being done, how and why, in the stages outlined in this and following chapters. Besides providing what, for most NHS managers, are unfamiliar technical skills such training can boost self-confidence and enable the marketing cycle to be completed faster than would otherwise occur. For middle and junior managers formal training is most suitable but for supervisors and non-managers the most suitable vehicle may be informal meetings or team briefing processes because they are interactive, allowing questions and doubts about an unfamiliar procedure to be aired.

Marketing as a means to quality assurance

Many NHS managers try to begin a marketing, or a quality assurance, project, by seeking a definition of service 'quality'. Most have already encountered some theoretical answers:

- Donabedian defines service quality as the balance of health benefits and harm produced by health care, to maximize which requires adequacy in process of care (monitored through clinical audit), structure (i.e. staffing levels and mix, managerial procedures, documentation) and in outcome.[2] However this definition mixes up the criteria of quality (outcome and elements of process) with the means to its achievement (structure and the other elements of process).
- Maxwell defines service quality as the possession of 'access to services, relevance to need (for the whole community), effectiveness (for individual patients), equity (fairness), social acceptability, and efficiency and economy'.[3] This conflates different agents' standpoints; the patient's, the buyer's and (if there is any such thing) society's.
- BS 4778 defines 'quality' as 'The totality of features and characteristics of a product or service which bear on its ability to satisfy a given need.'[4] For NHS purposes this needs a supplementary explanation of whose need and what these persons' needs for health services are.
- Crosby defines quality as 'conformance to requirements' but does not say (in the case of health services) whose requirements, or for what.[5]
- The US Joint Commission takes health service quality to consist of availability of care to the patients, identification of patient needs, timeliness of care, competence of staff, acceptability of care to the patient, minimizing patient risk, and ensuring a patient contribution to the health care process.[6]

To escape a purely conceptual debate about how to define 'quality' requires a definition open to practical, empirical interpretation. Of the above definitions the BSI's comes nearest to this. NHS marketing therefore requires the following definition of 'quality of a health service'.

Quality of a health service: the degree to which the service meets its users' instrumental needs for health care as these needs are revealed through empirical research.

Here health services are taken simply as 'instrumental' to meeting their users' needs for health and other needs, and users' demands are taken as the conscious expression (or misconception) of these needs.[7] On this view 'service quality' is defined not purely theoretically but largely empirically through a market research and the evaluation of services. The rest of the chapter shows how this can be done as part of the NHS marketing process.

Setting objectives and specifying quality through market research: an overview

The next two sections overview how market research and the evaluation of health services can be used to specify which services an NHS organization is to provide and to what quality. Figure 3.1 shows the main steps, their sequence and how they relate to NHS non-marketing activities (the same step numbers are used in the text). NHS managers are adopting the single term 'business planning' for the strategic planning of NHS buyers, sellers and directly-managed units. This convention is followed here, but reluctantly because it risks obscuring differences (explained below) in the marketing methods applicable to the different organizations in the internal market. Steps 1–6 in Figure 3.1 concern the buyer–seller interface (the internal market itself), steps 6–11 the marketing of a single department or service. (In the NHS the marketing of individual services is separated from, but presupposes, the earlier steps.)

The rationale for each step and the practicalities of applying them in an NHS organization are outlined below. This is followed by an explanation of outcome indicators. Chapter 4 explains how market research is undertaken for the various purposes mentioned in this chapter. Questions of which service to designate as non-core services, which core services to buy in rather than provide through directly managed units are addressed in Chapter 5.

'Business' planning in the NHS

Step 1. Establish prime objectives

Since NHS marketing is a technique for achieving its organizations' prime objectives, formulating them defines the ends to be served by market research and service evaluation, service design, promotional strategies, the choice of service mix and all other NHS marketing activities. Hence the business plan should list the prime objectives explicitly, ranked, with a specific deadline for achievement and where possible quantified. Some business plans add the rationale and benefit attaching to each objective. A business plan may list secondary objectives such as the desired public image and profile or which areas to attempt to become a technological leader and objectives for inter-sectoral planning. How prime objectives are formulated depends upon whether the organization is a seller.

For HAs, GPs and DMUs prime objectives would ideally be formulated

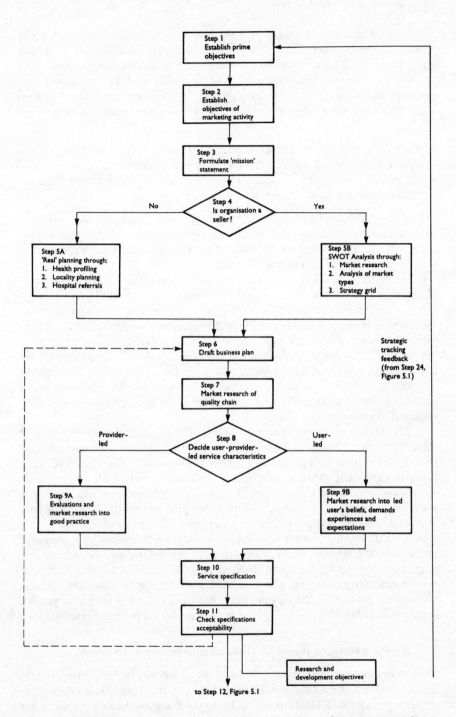

Figure 3.1 The NHS marketing process: objective and specification setting phases

in terms of quantified target populations, of the health status of these populations and of outcome indicators showing services' impact on health status (see pp. 73f.) and health behaviours (i.e. in real not financial terms). As yet few of these indicators are readily available to NHS managers but outcome indicators are so necessary to NHS marketing that the next section examines them more fully. Examples of objectives formulated in such terms might be:

- To reduce Neonatal Mortality Rate to 4.0 per 1000 live births whose obstetric care is provided by the DHA by 31 December 1992.
- To increase by 1% the proportion of stroke patients rehabilitated to a level where they can care for themselves at home.

In the absence of outcome indicators, service uptake and case mix, and some social indicators such as levels of sickness absence in the local labour force, are the only practically available (but very unsatisfactory) proxies for specifications of health status and outcome.

For sellers – SGTs, general practices selling subsidiary services, income-generating activities of HAs and DMUs – objectives are set in commercial terms of cash flow, 'surpluses' (i.e. profits; it appears that the Department of Health may set a permissible margin of ±6%), sales, market share and return on investment. Although rarely able to cost services on a per-item or per-patient basis, most NHS financial systems can already formulate objectives of this sort. But inexperience and gaps in NHS costing and pricing systems may lead the seller to overstate achievable profits. £250 000 profit sounds modest but at a 6% profit rate over £4 million turnover would be required to generate it.

Except where a completely new service is being commissioned many of the objectives will already be stated, or definable from, two main sources. Documentary sources such as *Working For Patients* and *Caring For People* give broad outlines, and other national policy documents such as *Maternity Care in Action* and *Health for All 2000*[8] more detailed objectives, as will the HA's annual and strategic programmes. Equally important practically is the *de facto* problem set; the legacy of existing services, the professions' concerns, managers' IPR and contract renewal agendas, the availability of money and the industrial relations climate constrain, or even determine, the substantive objectives. To recognize these aims among the stated objectives will help ensure that the marketing effort at least pursues organizationally realistic objectives. However the opportunity for critical and strategic objective setting will be under-exploited if the *de facto* problems predominate.

Step 2. Establish the objectives of marketing activity

From the organizational objective follow the objectives for marketing activities. Figure 3.2 shows the connections between marketing and other constituents of an NHS business plan. An explicit statement of objectives for marketing activity also defines:

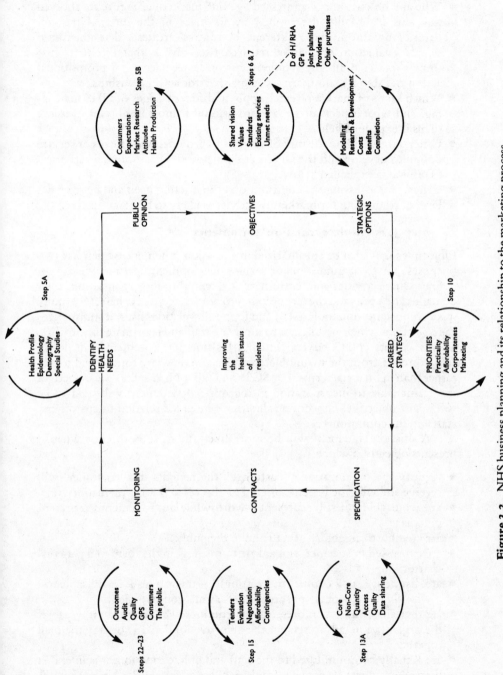

Figure 3.2 NHS business planning and its relationship to the marketing process

- Who are the 'customers' addressed by NHS marketing? Figure 2.1 showed that this is broadly determined by its place in the internal market. Prioritizing among these different 'customers' creates a decision-rule if service evaluation or market research later reveals that different 'customers' place conflicting requirements on service design or promotional activity. Table 3.1 summarizes the main customer relationships.
- Which kinds of market research apply to different stages of NHS marketing, and what aspects of service provision it is most important to track. (This is explained below.)
- Criteria for deciding the mix of services to provide, what forms of service design to develop and the targets and purposes of promotional activities. (This is also explained below.)
- Criteria for assessing the contribution of marketing itself and hence what level of resourcing for marketing activity is likely to be cost effective.

Step 3: Formulate 'mission' statements

Objectives may also be summarized in a mission statement, which has two purposes. Firstly it guides major service development decisions because it defines what activities and 'customers' are central to the organization, their demands and needs and the technologies to be used to satisfy these.[9] Secondly it is a communication tool to staff and for public relations uses. It summarizes the objectives which are likeliest to motivate staff and legitimate the organization's activity. NHS buyers' and DMUs' mission statements can derive fairly directly from the main objectives because these are formulated in real rather than in financial terms. For SGTs and other NHS sellers the objectives most amenable to incorporation in the mission statement will tend to be secondary objectives concerning the trust's intended relation to customers, staff and the community.

A mission statement will be more likely to serve both ends when it presents objectives which:

- identify the organization's 'customer', the benefits this 'customer' will receive and why the benefits offered by this organization are distinctive;
- are achievable but still represent a worthwhile improvement on present practice;
- are credible to all grades of staff and to the public;
- are expressed in succinct, sloganistic terms, e.g. in the form of a patients' charter;
- are distinctive (in a competitive setting)[10] – this makes it inadvisable too obviously to copy or adapt someone else's mission statement;
- are revisable to allow unforeseen opportunities to be added or (at worse) if the organization fails to achieve the objectives or decides to scrap them all together;
- are actually communicated to the staff and public to whom it is intended they communicate (not printed only in obscure internal documents such as the HAs annual programme);

Table 3.1 'Customer' relationships in the NHS internal market

Agent	Prime user	Secondary user	Paymaster	Other external publics	Internal publics
General Practice	Patients on GP list	Residential homes, HAs, employers, etc. for whom GP provides medical services, documentation, etc.	FHSA	Potential patients, informal carers	Support staff Other GPs in group practice or consortia
SHAs (except LPTHs)	DHAs, DMUs, SGTs	NHS employees	Department of Health via NHS Management Executive	Professional bodies, media, pressure groups	Staff, consultants, researchers
DHAs, RHAs, LPTHs (and equivalent in Wales, Scotland and N. Ireland)	Catchment population, including patients		Department of Health via NHS Management Executive	Mass media, pressure groups, Political publics	Employees
DMUs	Patients	GPs, care managers, tertiary referers	DHA, IG Activity, GPs with practice budget	Informal carers, workforces, employers	Employees
SGTs	Patients	GPs, care managers, tertiary referers	Buyers: DHA, RHA, insurers, individual patients, firms, GPs with practice budgets	Buyers Informal carers Workforces Employers	Employees
FHSAs	Resident population including patients		RHA	Mass media, pressure groups DHAs	Employees, committees

- are actually translated into action, i.e. the rest of the marketing process is implemented.

Mission statements are a method for organizational use. They are inapplicable, even ridiculous, in very small organizations such as the small general practice.

Step 4. Is the organization a seller?

Ordinarily this would be a straightforward factual question mentioned only for logical completeness. HAs, FHSAs, LAs and directly-managed units would answer 'no', SGTs would answer 'yes'. In respect of their marginal income-generating activities only, some general practices and DMUs would also answer 'yes'. Whether general practices would answer 'yes' in respect of primary care depends upon how far increasing the proportion of capitation fees in GP payments and relaxing controls on medical advertising actually has the intended effect of making GPs treat their patients as individual 'buyers'. Yet the question is fundamental because different forms of marketing apply to NHS buyers and directly-managed units (on the one hand) and to sellers (on the other).

The special circumstances of the NHS in the late 1980s make this a matter not of fact but of decision for NHS units: whether to seek self-governing trust status. Whether to become a competitor in the internal market is largely a marketing question. The decision depends on the answer to three questions.

The first is: would the proposed SGT be commercially viable? To find out one must answer a hypothetical 'yes' at step 5 and proceed to the market research outlined in step 6 (see p. 58). The hypothetical 'yes' can be made definite if, but only if, research confirms that all the following conditions hold:

- Buyers exist for the services the proposed SGT can offer.
- The services the SGT can offer are of a character and price that buyers wish to take or, in the case of case-cost or cost and volume contracts, are services that GPs wish to refer patients to.
- The relation between the scale of services buyers wish to buy, the costs to the SGT of providing them, and the price buyers are willing to pay is such as to put the SGT into profit.
- The proposed SGT could withstand competition from its main competitors and substitutes, including any potential new providers.
- Potential exists for the SGT to develop new services which also satisfy the above conditions.
- In the foreseeable future the above conditions are unlikely to change for the worse (from the SGT's viewpoint), for instance because of radically new health care technologies, major shifts in population or disease patterns, or changes in the buying organization.

By repeating these enquiries for different forms of the proposed SGT one can discover what services the SGT should include (e.g. whether it should be a fusion of previously separate units?). In deciding the size of an SGT it is also worth considering:

- Whether to include primary services (outreach clinics, screening services, etc.) that feed the main SGT services.
- Whether there are any other units with which the SGT now shares support services (e.g. laboratories), placing a one-unit SGT in a very strong (or very weak) commercial bargaining position because it monopolized (or lacked) support services originally provided District wide.
- Whether existing cross boundary flow towards the unit may suggest that an SGT would be able to supply several buyers.

The second question is whether the proposed SGT would be managerially viable. This depends upon whether the proposed SGT already has, or is confident it can acquire, the managerial capacity to undertake the marketing activities outlined in this and following chapters; depends, that is, on the findings of an audit of its probable marketing capacity.

Thirdly one must consider whether it is ethically and politically acceptable to seek SGT status. Many NHS chairmen and managers have experienced considerable covert political pressures to 'express interest' in SGT status. SGT status indeed offers unit level managers greater freedom from central over-control (particularly financial control). It may offer the medical and nursing professions an opportunity to reassert their power within the hospital polity. Against this must be weighed professional and public hostility towards 'opting out',[11] based upon the (well-founded) fear that becoming an SGT radically alters the purpose of providing health services in a commercial direction.

Step 5. Deciding service mix

Decisions on which service mix makes the greatest contribution to the objectives formulated at step 1 are made at this step. Here 'services' are defined as a strategic business unit or an (extended) 'product line'. A 'service' is defined in terms of buyers or of patient groups (defined by specialty, residence or referral route – e.g. as 'self-referred to family planning services') rather than by managerial function (i.e. as laboratory services, supplies, etc.) or by profession. The business plan lists the service it is intended to provide, and any significant omissions from that list. It is zero-based, not concerned only with the marginal year-on-year changes. Here too sellers and non-sellers differ.

Step 5A. For buyers and directly-managed units

Deciding what mix of services to provide resembles NHS planning of the middle 1980s in that decisions are made primarily by 'real', non-financial criteria (even if within cash limits; see step 11, p. 73) and differs from it in being zero-based. (This is rather far removed from 'business planning' in its usual commercial forms.) Ordinarily the plan will have to consider:

- The demographic and social mix of the total population served, hence which service mix gives most comprehensive health care cover (a predominantly elderly population is unlikely to need extensive maternity services). This also gives clues as to:
  - (i) The epidemiological character of the population, including their patterns of health behaviour (smoking, contraception, diet) and ill-health.
  - (ii) Their patterns of health service utilization, including balance between NHS and non-NHS service use, cross-boundary flows.
  - (iii) The scope for health maintenance and disease prevention, including intersectoral activities to influence the health impact of industries (e.g. chemical works, nuclear power installations) on their workers, their consumers and nearby residents. Past NHS planning and UK health policy has tended to under-rate this.
- The scale and character of the health service infrastructure and technologies likely to be available.

There are three main ways in which such planning can be undertaken (other texts elaborate).[12]

Health profiling is most relevant to geographically-based buyers, primary and community services, health promotion and general practice. A well-constructed health profile can give the NHS marketer critical information on the size, character and distribution of the population served and its main needs for preventive, primary and secondary services. Vignette 3.1 illustrates the content of one health profile. At HA level the task of constructing the necessary health profiles falls naturally to the DPH and specialists in community medicine. Health surveys serve the identical purpose.

Locality planning consists of designing a mix of services from public, commercial and informal sources to serve all the social care needs of the population of a given locality. From 1991 locality planning will be most relevant to DMUs in community mental illness services and the local authority purchasers of community care. It can be carried out at unit or sub-unit level (or the local authority equivalent) and is the organizational counterpart to care management. Locality planning is still in its infancy in many NHS community care services but many of the education centres are now disseminating practical knowledge of it.[13]

Hospital service mix would ideally also be derived from health profiles showing, from direct epidemiological research, the prevalence of conditions requiring secondary care in the target population. However, the underdevelopment of this type of health profiling in the NHS makes this generally unlikely in the near future. Deciding hospital service mix by projecting historical data on referral patterns and case mix, on the assumption that tertiary, GP and ambulance service referrals more or less reflect need for secondary health care, remains a defensible proxy. This proxy departs from

---

Vignette 3.1 Health profiling: an example

In 1984, the first Mersey Health Promotion Conference was held. To aid its deliberations a health profile of the region was produced. This excerpt from its contents pages indicates matters on which the profile presented data:

Defining the Problem
Years of Life Lost
The Determinants of Health
Health in Mersey; the Ecology of the Region
Geography
Circumstances of Life within the Region
The Black Report
The Population of Mersey Health Region
The Structure of the Population
Fertility within the Region
Abortion and Fertility
Infant Mortality
The Causes of Death and Ill-Health
Death in the Region
Causes of Death and Premature Years of Life Lost
Sickness and Ill-Health
    Secondary Care
    Primary Care
    Community Surveys
    Avoidable Deaths and the Quality of Medical Care

Source: Ashton, J *Health in Mersey, A Review*, Liverpool 1985 (Liverpool University, Department of Community Health).

---

the true profile to the extent that referral decisions are ill-judged or (much more importantly) insofar as people suffering from the condition in question either do not seek health care at all or present to someone other than an NHS GP.

Assuming that services will be bought from several sources, the HA will next have to decide how to divide its population into segments, each corresponding to a service contract. (A 'segment' is a sub-population of users having distinct needs and wants of the service, requiring a distinct service specification.) The planning data have now to be examined to discover what distinct sub-groups exist in population; what patterns in the demand and the need for health services are correlated with these sub-groups; and whether the differences in these patterns necessitate different specifications for health services for each sub-group. The answers determine whether a single specification can apply to the whole user population or a different specification is required for each user segment; and hence the minimum number of service contracts to draft.

NHS secondary services could be segmented by:

- Specialty or group of specialties. For planners this segmentation has the advantage of corresponding to existing NHS information categories and occupational demarcations. Segmentation by specialty simplifies contract drafting but there are few *a priori* grounds for thinking that patterns of patient demand or need correspond to specialty categories.
- Geography; a suitable segmentation where place of residence or travel patterns were closely correlated with health status or patterns of health service utilization.
- Care group. This segmentation is already familiar in the case of (e.g.) services for the elderly, maternity services or social care in the community for the mentally handicapped.
- By life cycle phase distinguishing services for young adults (emphasising trauma services, gynaecology, health promotion, etc.), for late-middle aged people (emphasizing cold surgery, rehabilitation, etc.), for mothers and children, for the elderly, etc.

The last two ways probably relate more closely to patterns of user need and demand than the first two. Many other ways of segmenting NHS services are imaginable. The Department of Health's apparent intention to press DHAs to fragment large block contracts[14] may encourage DHAs to explore these possibilities.

Step 5B. For sellers; SWOT analysis through market research

For sellers service mix is decided through a 'SWOT' analysis, a larger scale version of the same business planning (properly so called) as used in deciding on income-generating activities. In the NHS, SWOT analysis uses data produced by market research (Chapter 4 explains the methods) to assess:

- Competitors' strengths and weaknesses. 'Competitors' include producers of substitute services (e.g. 'alternative' and private medicine) as well as qualitatively similar services (e.g. other DGHs attracting cross-boundary flow of the local DGH's potential patients), potential new entrants to the markets as well as existing suppliers.[15]
- The relative commercial bargaining power of one's own organization against suppliers and buyers; is one able to dictate price and other contractual terms?
- Where does the service have competitive advantage or unique selling point (or the opposite)? In what ways is the service attractive (or repellent) to buyers and users?
- Potential size and profitability of different markets, and their main areas of growth and recession, possible areas for diversification in light of competitors' strengths and weaknesses.
- What obstacles (or opportunities) confront the expansion or redesign of services?

- Buyers' and users' beliefs about what services should be provided and what services are provided, and about providers' reputations.
- Sizes, profitability, stability of different markets and what prices the market can sustain.
- Ability to attract scarce resources, especially high-quality staff. This is less important than in the US system where hospitals try to attract physicians to seek admitting rights but NHS sellers may have to bear this in mind once they are allowed to offer differential rewards to such staff.

These market research data are then analysed in two main ways. One is an analysis of the market types confronting NHS sellers. NHS internal market buyer types will be:

- Statutory buyers (DHAs, RHAs, LAs, FHSAs) with large budgets and seeking broad population coverage, technically well informed about health services. For core services these buyers will be practically limited to HAs with whom there is already cross-boundary flow, but for non-core services this market could in principle include all buyers. Assuming continued under-funding of public health and social services, this is likely to start as a buyer's market. Such a large market will have many sub-segments (e.g. community, hospital and preventive services), each requiring its own analysis on the lines below.
- GPs with practice budgets, interested in clinical standards of staff and facilities, technical reputation, access and cost of services, well informed about health care, seeking a wide range of secondary services. This segment offers a large but very fragmented source of income. Once established it will probably be a comparatively stable market. (GPs without practice budgets count for marketing purposes as users not buyers of hospital services.)
- Health insurers, concerned with limiting per-case cost, seeking services with high presentational and 'hotel' standards, with high health expertise, seeking a narrow coverage (mainly cold surgery and occupational screening). This market is likely to grow intermittently under present health policy.
- Commercial buyers, usually employers with (in NHS terms) medium to small budgets, low expertise in health services, seeking a narrow coverage of services for staff to whom health care can be presented as a fringe benefit. This is likely to be a fluctuating market, following cycles in parts of the labour market outside the NHS. The same applies to the private medical market for NHS support services.
- Individual buyers have been a declining minority of private hospital customers since the middle 1970s and there seems little reason to doubt that this trend will continue.[16] (This is not to say that the sale of marginal 'extra' amenities to the users of free NHS hospital services will not increase in the short term.) The increased proportion of capitation fees in payments to GPs is intended to stimulate them to treat their patients as individual

buyers and most general practices have almost no other 'buyers'. This 'market' would be large but slowly growing.

Secondly a strategy for each of these market types, or for each major sub-segment of each market type, can then be inferred by applying the market research data to an appropriate business strategy grid. From such a grid the most profitable commercial strategy for each existing market, in the circumstances revealed by the market research results, can be read off or inferred. Table 3.2 summarizes the best-known grids. Kotler and Clarke's list curiously omits growing demand, unless this counts as 'latent'; but demand grows partly because buyers are aware, not unaware, of a new service they want. Their list is therefore modified for Table 6.2 to remedy this gap.

In choosing a grid it is worth considering:

- How closely each grid corresponds to the way in which the organization already understands its particular markets. In the NHS of the early 1990s this is likely to be decided negatively on the basis of which grid is least unfamiliar or unintelligible. Kotler and Clarke's list of demand patterns may appear least alien to the NHS because it was developed for health service use.[17]
- Is the data necessary to complete the grid available? In the existing state of NHS information systems this probably rules out all but the simplest grids (such as Boston) in the short term. Commercial confidentiality will also make some data (e.g. competitors' throughput) less accessible as the internal market develops.
- Degree of validation. However the most fully validated grid (PIMS) demands more market data to feed it than will be readily available to NHS managers in the near future.
- Can the grid be adapted? Grids developed for commercial uses, and even for the US health system, (e.g. Kotler and Clarke's) may require re-interpretation since it cannot be taken for granted that the market types found in a reimbursement funded health system will arise in NHS internal markets too. Standard grids may also require additions for NHS sellers' use. For instance a teaching hospital might also wish to consider which service mix offered the greatest clinical development and research opportunity.

The purpose of these analyses is to identify potentially profitable markets, whether the continuation of existing profitable services or the development of new services.

Step 6. Drafting the business plan

By their respective methods sellers and non-sellers can produce a business plan. Table 3.3 illustrates possible NHS business plan headings. Of greatest practical importance is that part of the plan dealing with implementation.

Table 3.2 Business strategy grid

Grid	Market type	Product type	Implied strategy	Information required
Boston	High growth	High market share ('star')	Maintaining or increasing market share	What extra marketing support required? What potential to become 'star'?
		Low market share (problem child)	Up or out: increase market share or drop the product	
	Low growth	High market share (cash cow)	Keep market position; Reinvest to maintain/aid growing SBUs	Market shares. Growth potential for SBUs
		Low market share ('dog')	Reduce or abandon	—
PIMS	Any	High market share compared with three main competitors High value added Comparatively high quality product Easy to innovate and differentiate Vertically integrated production	Invest and develop; tailored reports provided by (US) Strategic Planning Institute	PIMS database
		Other	Defend market share or withdraw	
	High industry growth	Any	Invest and develop tailored reports provided by (US) Strategic Planning Institute	

Table 3.2 *continued*

Grid	Market type	Product type	Implied strategy	Information required
Product/ Opportunity	Old	Old	Increase market penetration	How to attract new customers?
		New	Product development	Possible minor product developments
	New	Old New	Market development Diversification	Possible new product uses Possible new markets
Modified Kotler and Clarke	Third-party payer, Charitable, Cash and Carry	Negative demand (i.e. willingness to pay not to use a service)	Offer insurance or preventive services	Market share, sales trends, ratio of supply to demand
		Latent demand	Create knowledge of the services/product	
		Falling demand	Defend market share	
		Irregular demand		
		Full demand	Defend market share or withdraw	
		Overfull demand		
		Unwholesome demand	Withdraw	
		Growing demand	Invest	
General Electric	Highly attractive	High business strength Middle business strength Low business strength	Invest and grow Invest and grow Selectivity and earning	Market attractiveness depends on: Size of markets Stability markets Level of competition Capital intensity Economies of scale Likelihood of technical innovations

			Business strengths depend on:
Middle attractiveness	High business strength	Invest and Grow	Product with differential advantage
	Middle business strength	Selectivity and earning	
	Low business strength	Harvest/divest	
Low attractiveness	High business strength	Selectivity and earning	Sales values
	Middle business strength	Harvest/divest	Sales growth
	Low business strength	Harvest/divest	Possible product ranges
			Management of sales and distribution
			Price level controllable
			Profit level controllable
			Innovativeness of time
			Able to exploit economics of scale
Porter Generic Strategy Model			
Broad target for competitive scope	Low cost	Cost leadership – mass production and low cost	Market shares, competitor analysis
	Differentiated	Differentiation of product price less important, build brand loyalty	
Narrow target for competitive scope	Low cost	Cost focus – niche or specialist pricing	
	Differentiated	Differentiation focus niche/specialist product design	

Table 3.3   Possible headings in an NHS business plan

Objectives
   Health objectives
   Commercial objectives

The Environment
   Demographic and epidemiological trends
   Changes in health service organization and technology
   Legal and regulatory changes
   National trends in spending on health services

The main markets served: for each of these
   Who the buyers are; the main markets and their segments
   Who the users are, and their main segments
   Changes in market size and buyer demands
      Potential new markets
      Declining or endangered markets
   Existing service provision
   Areas of strength – competitive and bargaining advantages
   Areas of weakness – their causes and implications
   Reputation of the service with buyers and users
   Strategy for the plan period
   Changes in health behaviours, referral patterns and user demands
   Assumptions on which the forecast and strategy rest

Competitors
   Who the main competitors are (NHS and non-NHS)
   Potential new competitors
   Competitors' strengths and weaknesses
   Strengths and weaknesses of own marketing activities

Implementation
   Main targets and time scales
   Lead responsibilities
   Development of new services

From this, and from earlier parts of the plan, the responsible managers have to be able to read off for the service they manage the:

- Target populations – which may be defined by clinical specialty, place of residence or work, or referral pattern.
- Format – whether to provide the service on an in-patient, day-patient or out-patient basis, institutionally or in the community.
- Utilization – volume of uptake or throughput, broad case mix, the referral routes into the service and the discharge routes out.
- The service infrastructures (laboratories, CSSD, estates, patient information, etc.) required to support the chosen service mix.
- Overall human resources (mix, skills)
- Overall cost and, for sellers, sales, income and profit.
- Positioning against competitors. It is obviously important for sellers but DHAs and DMUs also need to decide whether to co-operate with private

medicine or to incorporate 'alternative' medicine. It is worth considering whether other providers offer complementary services to the NHS, with potential for co-operation and cross referral.

- Assumptions as to changes in uptake, technology, social and political setting, epidemiology. These must be stated explicitly so that any predictive errors can later be diagnosed.
- Main implementation deadlines, reporting arrangements, control and review processes, including (for present purposes) who is to carry out the remaining steps in the marketing process.
- Key variables (e.g. utilization, outcomes, quality; explained below) for tracking.

These objectives for each service then have to be checked for mutual consistency, comprehensiveness, and that the implied total levels of cost, throughput, etc. add up to the whole-organizational totals decided at step 1. The resulting 'business' plan sets the framework for the remaining stages of NHS marketing. These are repeated for each service and begin with the setting of a service specification.

Setting service quality specifications through evaluation and market research

Step 7. Market research into the quality chain

Now the marketer focuses on the individual service and its users. Depending on the type of service, the patient or the target population is taken as the prime 'user' with, for hospital services, the GPs as the ancillary 'user'. For sellers in the NHS internal market this is a shift of focus from the buyers' demands that preoccupied the previous steps.

The term 'quality chain' has been coined[18] to describe the whole process in which a user comes into contact with a health service during an episode of health care, crossing organizational boundaries during the experience and continuing his or her other activities as well as he or she can meanwhile. Step 7 is to reconstruct this chain empirically, through market research to discover what actually happens to the users during their contact with the service. The purpose is to discover what aspects of the service's interaction with the users it is necessary to manage, and how, in order to meet the provider's prime objectives. The main dimensions of the users' experience it is necessary to examine are:

- Points at which the user's choice determines whether the service is used and in what way (e.g. the patient's initial decision to seek medical advice, or his compliance with the treatment plan).
- The 'core product' i.e. the broad types of care provided, their expected outcomes and risks, and the 'peripheral products' (e.g. booking arrangements, hotel services, that only support it).

- Practical contributions made to care by family, friends and other informal carers, and by other organizations.
- Social character of the episode (e.g. who the patient meets, the contrasting social roles adopted by patients and NHS staff).
- Psychological character of the episode for the patient (e.g. what anxieties do patients feel? what reassurances do they seek?)
- The information flows between patient and the NHS, the ways in which this information is elicited, communicated and recorded, and how accurately.
- For sellers, knowledge of the money flows resulting from the episode and the associated administrative procedures (methods for claiming payment etc.) is critical.
- Physical location of the events and the transport implications of this, the 'hotel' facilities and any clinical equipment which the patient encounters.
- Points at which the provider's decision determines whether the service is used and in what way (e.g. the doctor's decision whether to refer a patient to hospital or another agency).
- Whether the first seven of the above factors differ markedly between different sub-groups within the target population.
- The profile of the user population in terms of its age, sex, occupational, ethnic, geographic and any other characteristics which may provide a clue to possible segmentation (see below). If this personal data is not collected at this stage it becomes difficult or impossible to segment the user population later.

It is necessary to identify the 'critical points' which have the greatest impact upon whether, or how far, the user's and the provider's objectives are met. How detailed this reconstruction of users' experience of the service has to be depends upon how closely defined the quality standards and service design are to be (see below).

Figure 3.3 shows a worked example of an acute out-patient episode.

Step 8. Decide user-led and provider-led service characteristics

The step determines which service standards are to be determined (vicariously) by the service user through market research and which by the provider through technical evaluation (including clinical and epidemiological evaluation). This allocation is not an arbitrary management choice.

User-led service characteristics can be categorized according to whether they are:

- Necessarily user-led – these are the service characteristics influencing those user behaviours which in turn determine whether the NHS organization achieves its objectives, and in which the user acts largely autonomously of the NHS. For out-patient services an example would be the characteristics determining GP's choice of hospital to refer to (say the clinical reputation

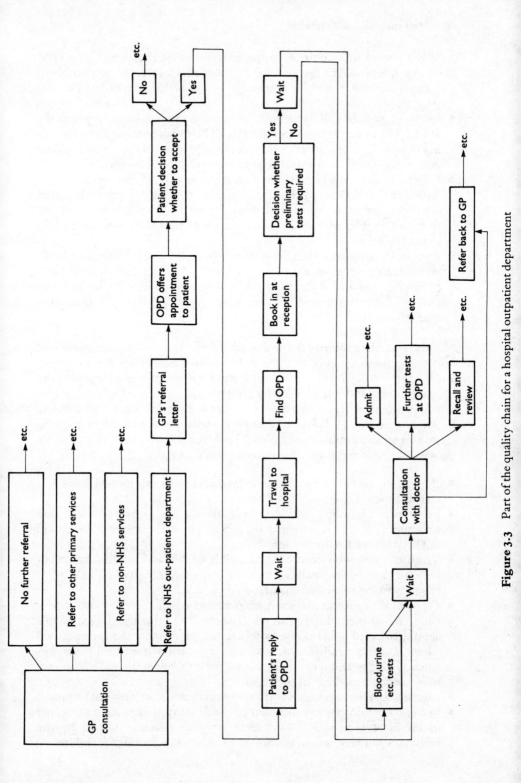

Figure 3.3 Part of the quality chain for a hospital outpatient department

of the consultants or the existence of a specialized resource). For GPs, an example would be the practice characteristics which decide a patient to sign up for that particular practice (e.g. the availability of late evening surgeries).

- User-led by policy, for example the location of non-core services or the availability of extra 'amenities' for sale to NHS hospital patients, according to *Working for Patients*.[19] These can be read off from the relevant policy documents which will already be familiar to NHS managers.
- Rationally user-led because they concern aspects of the service about which the user knows best. One example is what clinical information a patient wishes to know and what forms of presenting it he or she finds intelligible; another is the suitability of secondary services to GPs requirements.
- Optionally user-led – with these aspects of the service it is arguable either way whether the providers or the users know best what service standards to set but a policy decision is taken, supererogatorily, to let the user choose. Examples would include allowing patients access to their own medical records.

Market research to identify the necessarily user-led service characteristics and how they influence user behaviours and decision is non-optional in principle, and for present-day NHS managers practically non-optional in regard to the characteristics which are user-led by policy.

Depending on circumstances, provider-led service characteristics may be determined by a DMU or SGT autonomously, or stipulated by a buyer as terms of a service contract and thus adopted by the DMU or SGT providing the service. Provider-led service characteristics are those:

- Beyond the user's technical knowledge or expertise to select. Most clinical technicalities of diagnosis and treatment fall into this category.
- Preventing ill health, and detecting or treating presymptomatic and asymptomatic disease, of which the user will by definition be unaware and unlikely to seek health care for.
- Treating users who need but are unable to demand health care, either because of ill health itself, or they are too young or have no relative or friend who can reliably demand it on their behalf.
- Over which different service users' interests conflict, for instance where children and their elderly parents disagree as to whether ill aged people should be cared for at home or where the buyer's and the (prospective) users' interests conflict, e.g. when government wishes health services (such as the provision of contraception for girls below the age of consent) to be used as a medium of social control.[20]
- Meeting legal requirements and the requirements of professional ethics.
- In respect of which user beliefs and demands are systematically misformed in an ideological way;[21] a widely-accepted example would be the Jehovah's Witness' refusal to consent to blood transfusions for children.

Table 3.4 User- and provider-led elements of the quality chain shown in Figure 3.3: a worked example

Provider-led characteristics	*User-led characteristics*
Acceptance of GP's referral	*Necessarily user-led*
Decision of which doctor and other staff to see and treat patient	GP decision to refer to OPD
Choice of preliminary clinical tests	Patient decision to accept OPD appointment
What TP to offer	Consent to treatment plan (TP)
Safety and competence standards for clinical procedures	Compliance with TP
Completion of any legally required consents, ensuring that patient consent is informed consent	Relatives' or informal carers' assistance with TP
Decision whether to refer to other agencies, to offer hospital admission or refer back to GP	*User-led by policy*
	Length of wait for OPD appointment
	Length of wait at OPD
Decision of what clinical outcome can reasonably be expected in the circumstances	Availability of shop, refreshments, telephone and other facilities at OPD
	Rationally user-led
	Appointment date and time
	Advance information of access to OPD, likely course of events, etc.
	Details to be given of the illness or condition and its treatment
	Furnishing and ambience of OPD buildings
	Staff manner and attitudes

As a corrective to the alleged bureaucratization and professionalization of the NHS it might be argued that when it is doubtful whether a service standard should be set by users or providers the onus of proof should lie with those who allege the providers should set it; but such a case can often be made. Table 3.4 continues the previous worked example.

Step 9. Setting quality specifications

Specifications (or 'standards') for provider-led and for user-led service characteristics are set by different methods.

Step 9A. Provider-led standards

In provider-led aspects of the service, standards can be set by reference to 'good practice': 'good' in the sense of 'meeting organizational objectives'. What is 'good practice' depends upon whether the organization is a seller. For non-sellers good practice is defined in real, technical terms. For sellers 'good practice' is what suffices to out-compete other sellers commercially. 'Good practice' can be discovered from three main sources:

- Market research into existing best practice elsewhere, especially competitors (Chapter 4 explains possible market research methods), to discover what forms of service prove successful in attracting patients or cash or in enhancing the reputation of (other) health services and to find out what new forms of service are under development. Innovations often begin at margins of the health system, making it worth investigating not only the established research centres and teaching hospitals but 'alternative' and commercial medicine, overseas health systems, voluntary services and developmental work by suppliers to the NHS (e.g. in the fields of pharmaceuticals, prosthetics). Competitors' practice demonstrates what service standards are not only technically, but organizationally achievable. In practice much of this has to be done from secondary sources but it may be feasible for health managers to observe some alternative forms of service at first hand.

- Technical evaluations include clinical trials and experimental projects reported in the academic, clinical and professional journals. They show technically achievable levels of outcome and the associated risks and side-effects of different patterns of care, and incidentally give clues as to which outcome indicators are clinically pertinent (see below). Comparison of local with national figures for the few national outcome-monitoring systems such as CEPOD can be used to discover mean and best levels achieved in normal service conditions. In practice most evaluative data will have to be obtained from secondary sources. The obvious people to undertake both this work, and direct evaluative studies, are the appropriate clinical heads of service and (in HAs) the Directors of Public Health and their staff; if there is any justification for involving clinicians in management it is for such purposes.
- National policy and advice from the Department of Health, the Royal Colleges and other professional bodies, from pressure and other interest groups (e.g. MIND, ASH), and from defence organizations, legal advisers and other monitoring bodies such as the Health and Safety Executive. At one extreme of standard-setting these bodies can advise on the legally and ethically acceptable minima for standards of service. At the other they recommend preferable new forms of service.

Step 9B: User-led standards

User-led standards can be discovered from service users themselves using the market research methods outlined in the next chapter. The same questions have to be asked of potential users when user-led service characteristics are being specified for new or expanded services. For setting user-led standards market research addresses three questions:

- What characteristics do users want of the service – and which of these are the critical characteristics determining the user's decision to use or refuse the services? The answer to this question determines what aspects of the service users most want standards set for.
- What do users perceive as the salient characteristics of existing services, and how do they compare with the characteristics users want?
- Against what standards or points of comparison do service users implicitly

judge local services (e.g. do they implicitly compare hospital out-patient areas with hotel reception areas? With an airport lounge? With a service station?)

Then service standards are simply 'read off' from the results of the market research. If for instance clinic users think a wait of over 15 minutes after appointment for the doctor is unacceptable but would prefer no delay at all, and if it has been decided that the users know best about acceptability of waiting times, then there is the service standard for maximum permissible delay ready-made.

Step 10. Producing the service specification

To produce the service specification from the above data involves deriving suitable formulations for the service standards. The finished service specification combines user-led with the provider-led standards. At least the standards relating to critical points identified at step 7 must be included and the number of key standards must be small enough to allow management and tracking not to be overwhelmed by comparatively unimportant detail. It is prudent to specify the service in greater detail for the important specifications, i.e. where:

- There is potential conflict of interests between HAs and providers e.g. when achievement (or non-achievement) of a given standard triggers payment (or non-payment). The more closely a service contract resembles a standard commercial contract the greater the potential for such conflicts.
- For aspects of service with potentially far-reaching consequences for the patient or the organization (e.g. on patient safety, confidentiality of medical information)
- Detailed tracking is necessary for legal, ethical or technical-evaluative reasons
- There are reasons to expect that the provider may have difficulty sustaining the stipulated standard in practice, for instance when a new service specification departs from previously accepted practice.

Table 3.5 illustrates some ways in which standards for the main characteristics of a NHS in-patient service might be formulated, and criteria for deciding the key standards to monitor services by and (in the case of HAs) to select possible providers by.

It is prudent to supplement service specifications used as the basis for a service contract with provision for negotiation on minor points not anticipated at the outset. For tracking purposes (see Chapter 5) the minimum tolerable levels of achievement against the specification must also be decided for the main indicators. These minima will act as 'trigger points' for more detailed tracking, other investigations, or even contract renegotiation if the provider fails to satisfy them. The service specification may be presented in the form of a prospectus or 'service manual'. Chapter 5 explains how the specification becomes the basis of a service contract.

Table 3.5 Formulating service quality specifications

Aspect of service	Form of indicators	Criteria for selecting key indicator
Outcome Survival Function Pain Morale	Outcome indicators	Amenability to health service influence Clinical pertinence Patient preferences
Normalization of social life	Outcome indicators Destination on discharge As determined by MR into patient preferences	Patient preferences 'Good practice' Health policy
Participation in own health care Health maintenance Health behaviours	Prevalence of obesity, smoking exercise, alcohol consumption, etc.	WHO *HFA 2000*
Health education/informatics	Scored levels of user knowledge of health behaviours and risks	National Policy WHO targets Epidemiological pertinence
Preventive care	Uptake of vac. and imm., family planning, ante-natal care, GP care, dentistry, services, etc.	
Appropriate treatment and care Appropriateness of diagnostic methods and TP	Existence of process for checking (e.g. clinical audit) 'Cookbooks' – list of acceptable/reimbursable procedures	Technical availability Implementability Clinical pertinence

Iatrogenesis	Avoidable deaths	Clinical pertinence
	Cross infection	National policy
	Unintended returns for treatment	Seriousness and possible risk to patients
	Incidence of complaints, litigation	
Personalized care, Individualized		
Staff behaviours	Observation checklist	
Clinical Information: Availability Intelligibility	Response rates to surveys	Patient preference as revealed by MR
Patient satisfaction with: Staff manner Privacy Choice of ADL	Response rates and surveys	Patient preference as revealed by MR
Patient morale, autonomy	Outcome indicators	Clinical pertinence, Good practice
Choice		
Range of services available to patient	Checklist	National policy business plan
Alternative patterns of care	Checklist	National policy, business plan
Patient awareness of available services	Patient knowledge rates of range of services	National policy, business plan
Environment of NHS care		
Ambience/atmosphere	Response rates to MR of patient opinions	Patient preferences
Appearance Cleanliness Tidiness Light	Observation checklist Measurement	Patient preferences Legal and building regulations standards

Table 3.5 *continued*

Aspect of service	Form of indicators	Criteria for selecting key indicator
Safety	Satisfactory to third party	As stated by law, fire regulations, etc.
Warmth	Direct measurement	Patient preference
Access		
Waiting times	Times	Patient preferences
Transport times		National policy/standards
Opening hours		
Availability of services	See above	
Availability of creche/care for dependants	Checklist	
Waiting areas, information refreshments, etc. for relatives/friends.	Checklist	

The headings in the 'Aspect of service' column are taken from *Working For Patients* and supporting documents, and from *Health for All 2000*. For these purposes many outcome indicators are best formulated in probabilistic terms, for instance as: 'There will be a 98% recovery rate without complications for surgical procedure X' (see p. 75). The term 'clinical pertinence' is borrowed from US hospital quality assurance and means that the outcome indicators that clinical practice relies on most heavily should be the key specifications for clinical aspects of the service. 'Alternative patterns of care' are those choices shown by market research to be practically meaningful to patients (e.g. degree of invasiveness rather than the choice of formulation of tablets). This range of choice is obviously limited by the clinical technologies available; alternative forms of (say) contraception are technically available but not alternative methods of treating acute appendicitis. 'Patient preferences' are those service characteristics which market research at step 9B showed patients attach the greatest importance to in deciding whether to in deciding whether to use a particular health service.

Step 11. Check specification acceptability

Before it can be implemented, the service specification must be checked for consistency with the 'business' plan. Although an NHS service specification abstracts from all of the following factors (except perhaps utilization levels, and price in the case of services sold directly to the public) it has implications for the 'business' plan objectives in respect of:

- Cost; indeed without a service specification it is difficult to produce accurate, detailed service costings for business planning purposes.
- Utilization levels; the desired level of utilization, combined with a budget for providing the service, places a cost limit on the specification that can be adopted.
- Efficiency levels; service specifications define the outcome side of cost–benefit analyses, cost-efficiency analyses and other efficiency calculations.
- Income; which depends upon whether the buyers are able and willing to meet the costs of the specified service; in the case of sellers, profitability also depends upon this.
- Implementability, in particular whether the service specification is likely to be acceptable to staff and whether the providing organization has the managerial capacity to implement it. Buyers should beware of setting service quality specifications so high that providers will not risk tendering for the work.
- Achievability of the prime objectives. Service specifications are derived from 'best practice' on the above model but there is no guarantee that this is good enough to achieve the organization's prime objectives. If not, the major shortfalls between the prime objectives and what is technically achievable indicates the main areas for research and development activities. Meanwhile the service specification offers the best currently achievable standards.

In practice difficulties are likeliest to arise over the question of whether the specification can be provided within the cost limits required by the business plan.

If the service specification proves incompatible with the 'business' plan on any of these counts Step 6 and perhaps even some of the consequent evaluation and market research may have to be repeated until a service specification compatible with the 'business' plan emerges. Then the NHS marketing process can continue to the steps described in Figure 5.1 and Chapters 5 to 6.

Specifying clinical outcomes

Uses of outcome indicators

Of the standards required for specifying NHS services for marketing and quality assurance purposes clinical outcome indicators are currently the least familiar to NHS managers. US quality assurance and accreditation procedures are gradually focusing less on resources and more upon outcome. Whilst the content and sources will obviously differ, similar principles for selecting, inventing and applying indicators apply to other dimensions of service quality. Without outcome indicators there is little rational basis for determining the impact of health services upon their recipients' health, for evaluating new forms of care, for indicating the effectiveness in cost–benefit and cost effectiveness analyses and when determining ethical and legal claims or principles, for deciding treatment plans or for determining the *prima facie* appropriateness of diagnosis, treatment and care in clinical audit.

Types of outcome indicator

The many existing outcome indicators can be categorized in several dimensions. Which outcome indicator is best suited to marketing or quality assurance in a particular service depends partly upon where the indicator stands in these five dimensions:

- *Profiles vs. indices.* A profile itemizes many different constituents of health status separately and provides an independent measure of each. For instance, the Nottingham Health Profile separately deals with a patient's sleeping patterns, pain, mobility, morale, home life and other aspects of daily functioning.[22] Indices offer a single measure of health status. The various severity indicators with which many US health services now supplement DRGs allocate a patient's condition to a single category (e.g. Computerized Severity Index, APACHE II)[23] For NHS managers QALYs are probably the best-known attempt to produce a common outcome indicator for all services.
- *Level of generality.* Indicators have been developed which deal with the mortality of whole populations (e.g. SMRs, survival rates), with their morbidity (e.g. indicators of the incidence and prevalence of disease), with the health of the individual person (e.g. the Sickness Impact Profile),[24] with one particular function (e.g. rheumatological indicators of mobility,[25] attempts to produce indicators of pain),[26] or at a systemic and biochemical levels (e.g. white blood cell count, xenon clearance). Some indicators include the duration of changes in outcome or the urgency of need for care e.g. the indices developed by Karnofsky, Barthel, Grogona and Woodgate, and Spitzer.[27]
- *Aspect of health care.* Indicators have been developed to indicate physical outcome (e.g. severity indices), outcome in terms of the social setting produced for a client or patient (e.g. the Index of Adult Autonomy) and of the living environment (e.g. the Revised Resident Management Practice Scale[28]), psychological outcome (e.g. Rosow Morale Scale[29]), for behavioural and functional outcomes (e.g. the Isaac-Walkey Mental Status Score).[30] Some indicators combine several aspects (e.g. the Nottingham Health Profile).
- *Direct vs. proxy indicators.* Some indicators attempt a direct indication of health, an approach most evident in indicators developed for clinical use

such as the Apgar scale. Others offer a proxy by indicating the state of a variable such as ability to work or immunized status believed to be correlated with health (either as a cause of health status, as in the case of immunization, or an effect of it, as in the case of sickness absence from work). The Therapeutic Intervention Severity Scale takes the complexity of clinical intervention indicated as a proxy for severity of condition,[31] smoking might be taken as a behavioural proxy for risk of premature death through cardiovascular disease.[32] How valid an indicator of health such a proxy is depends upon how strongly this causal connection or correlation holds.

- *Probabilistic vs. absolute indicators.* Probabilistic terms are used to formulate some outcome measures (e.g. 5-year survival rates), others are in absolute terms (e.g. vision test scores).

Sources of outcome indicators

Because outcome indicators are so little used in most areas of NHS management, NHS management documents are usually a barren source of outcome indicators. However the main alternative sources are less easily accessible to NHS managers. Some provide empirical indications of health status but most only suggest what outcome indicators might be used, leaving the collection of data to the NHS marketer. They include:

1 Clinicians themselves will know any outcome indicators already used by clinicians in judging the outcome for individual patients or, for example, clinical trials but not yet collated for the service as a whole. They may also be able to advise on:

- Clinical literature – this is large and diverse but parts can be searched automatically via such databases as the DHSS database, Medline or Current Contents. Database searches can be arranged via medical and university libraries, but these searches yield only publication titles or (sometimes) abstracts and have to be followed up by consulting the research articles themselves.
- WHO publications, especially the appendices to *Health For All 2000*, use outcome indicators (sometimes proxy indicators) to formulate WHO policy objectives but in principle the same indicators can also be applied to other uses.[33]
- Professional bodies' publications and policy recommendations sometimes include key outcome indicators. For example, professional bodies' activities in the area of outcome assessment include the confidential inquiries into deaths occurring in hospital (CEPOD, The Confidential Enquiry into Maternal Deaths). Early in 1990 work was in hand to extend these inquiries beyond surgery and obstetrics. Whilst these sources tend to respect professional rather than patient demarcations and interests, organizations such as the Kings Fund can take a wider view.

2 Directories and other healthcare marketing literature. Directories of

outcome and quality indicators are still few and cover social, community and long-term care rather than acute care.[34] Vignette 3.2 reproduces one such directory entry. The lack of a similar directory for acute care is a major gap in current health service management research. Directories of quality assurance activities[35] may provide an indirect route to further outcome indicators via interested individuals. There are a few general texts on outcome indicators, and the burgeoning quality assurance literature.[36]

3 Health economists have attempted to develop outcome indicators but the best known (QALYs) has serious limitations (see below) and was developed more to give economic orthodoxy some purchase on non-commercial NHS practice than as a means of managing service quality.[37] A

Vignette 3.2   The autonomy scale

An extract from a recent index of outcome and process indicators.
Authors: Baker, B. L., Seltzer, G. B. and Seltzer, M. M.
Date: 1977
Purpose
The scale was developed in a study of community residences for mentally-retarded adults in the USA. It was designed to measure the extent to which restrictions were imposed upon the activities of people living in these residences.
Content
The scale consists of four items covering policy concerning entertaining the opposite sex, alcohol use within the residence, the curfew times and rules relating to bedtimes.
Administration
The items comprising this scale were incorporated in a questionnaire which was completed by heads of establishments who received the questionnaire through the post. The items are rated in terms of the presence or absence of restrictions and the type of restriction where restrictions operate. The percentage of areas in which restrictions operate is obtained by summing the responses to the items.

   Completion of the items requires no special training. No indication of the time taken to complete these items is given.
Scientific credibility
Standardisation   No research data are available.
Reliability   No research data are available.
Validity   The measure clearly differentiated between different kinds of residences for retarded adults operating in the community in the United States. Autonomy being found to be highest in semi independent community residences.

References
Baker, B. L., Seltzer, G. B., Seltzer, M. M. (1977) *As Close As Possible*. Boston, Little Brown.

Source: Raynes, NV, *Annotated Directory of Measures of Environmental Quality for Use in Services for People with a Mental Handicap*, Manchester 1988 (Manchester University Department of Social Policy and Social Work) pp. 14–5.

few of the economic studies in such journals as the *Journal of Health Economics* occasionally include their own outcome indicators.

4 Non-NHS bodies collect data which indicate health outcomes in broad terms. Data on absence from work, registered disability, destination on discharge from hospital, industrial injuries, RTAs, etc. are available but the sources are scattered. They include local authorities, the Health and Safety Executive, the police, Department of Social Security and voluntary agencies such as MIND. OPCS data is rich and detailed but collected too infrequently (decennially) to be of use in monitoring the outcome of any but the longest-term health programmes.

5 Epidemiological indicators such as data on SMRs, LEB and notifiable diseases can sometimes be obtained from the Department of Health, Regional Health Authority or the OPCS.

6 Patients or carers can themselves assess certain aspects of outcome (e.g. pain control, ability to carry on activities of everyday living). The market research methods outlined in the next chapter can be used to identify possible indicators and collect corresponding data.

7 Official inquiries such as the Short report[38] sometimes use outcome indicators but (because they usually concern issues at national level) often at a high degree of aggregation and over a long period.

8 Overseas practice, especially American since the US health system much influenced *Working for Patients*,[39] also suggests possible outcome indicators. However, use of outcome indicators in the US system appears to be oriented mainly towards risk management (to minimize costs of litigation) rather than towards assessing positive outcomes of health care. The accreditation manuals are of limited help.

What to look for in selecting an outcome indicator

Having found possible outcome indicators it is necessary to select those most valid (see the first six points in the following list), appropriate to the marketing needs of the service, and reliable. The sources of the outcome indicator should next be checked for evidence as to how far the candidate indicator:

- Is at the relevant level of generality, covering all the relevant aspects of outcome ('content validity').
- Is of the appropriate degree of certainty. Absolute indications of outcome are appropriate for setting legal and safety standards (e.g. that no one should die through anaesthetic mistakes). More probabilistic indicators may be appropriate for monitoring positive outcomes of care since the outcome of a treatment can seldom be guaranteed. The more standardized the treatments of a patient group the easier it is to develop, compare and aggregate outcome indicators ('cookbook medicine' is the extreme case) and the more applicable do absolute indicators become.
- Yields readings consistent with those given by other indicators when applied to the same patients or population ('criterion-related validity').

- Is plausible to its users, especially clinicians, as an indicator of outcome ('face validity').
- Is 'clinically pertinent' i.e. an indicator likely to be acceptable and widely useful to practitioners (besides marketers) in managing individual patients and case mix.
- Rests on defensible factual assumptions, if it is a proxy indicator ('internal validity'). If, for instance, an index has been standardized one must check what assumptions about possible confounding factors have been made, and whether other factors which might distort comparisons (e.g. occupational mix besides sex and age) have also been taken into account in the combination rules.
- Is precise and sensitive; able to discriminate changes of the degree likely to result from the marketing strategy but also insensitive to irrelevant influences. For instance, mortality data indicate the effect of all causes of reductions in deaths not only the impact of health services. The most suitable outcome indicator is the one most sensitive to the factors the health organization intends to influence through its marketing work.
- Makes no normative assumptions, but failing that states them explicitly. For instance QALYs and life-years saved implicitly favour treatment of the younger patient. The weighting systems used to summarize various more detailed indicators into summary single-measure indicators (in the narrow sense, as opposed to profiles) are often a source of bias. Mistakes here can lead into deep ethical and legal water. Some early work on weighting QALYs gave some outcomes a *negative* QALY value,[40] implying (if one accepted QALYs) a policy of passive euthanasia.
- Is reliable, i.e. produces consistent readings for the same patient's or population's condition when applied by different observers. Reliability is important when information systems rely on comparatively unskilled data collectors as is the case for much routinely collected and marketing data.
- Is reducible, i.e. capable of being aggregated and disaggregated into outcome indicators of lower or higher generality. Reducibility firstly provides a mutually coherent set of outcome indicators for different levels of management, and between indicators for managerial, clinical and epidemiological use. QALYs, for example, are reducible because outcome statements in terms of QALYs are logically equivalent to (much more complicated) statements about the relative preferences that specified individuals attach to different combinations of pain and disability.[41]
- Uses already available data, or requires data which is simple and cheap to collect accurately and reliably by comparatively untrained staff. One should consider whether the data can be processed through standard software such as SPSS and whether data formulated using the indicator can be (or needs to be) standardized for case mix or the mix of ages, sexes or DRGs.

Inventing an outcome indicator

Since the development of outcome indicators is uneven and many existing indicators do not satisfy all of the above criteria, it may often be necessary to devise a new outcome indicator for a particular service. The main steps are:

1 Identify the marketing decisions which it is intended to make, using information formulated through the indicator. These decisions determine what changes in outcome the indicator is required to indicate, the level of generality required and what aspects of the service are to be covered. For instance to decide what forms of treatments for varicosity to offer might require indicators of patient mobility, pain, probability of the varicosity recurring and risks of iatrogenesis.

2 Devise a candidate outcome indicator. Clinical practice is a useful starting point. Clinicians may already use implicit, but only partly articulated, indications of outcome in deciding when to discharge and in judging whether a patient episode went well or badly. A clinically pertinent outcome indicator will then be one which formulates these clinical intuitions explicitly. Existing indicators in other areas of care may suggest analogies or provide models.

3 If an index not a profile is required, rules need to be devised for combining and weighting the constituent indicators which the index is to summarize. Three methods are widely used. Reduction consists of defining points on the index as logically equivalent to a set of more concrete statements. For example the second of four points points one severity scale is defined as: 'Problems limited to an organ or system; significantly increased risk of complications [e.g.] . . . pyephlebitis with or without liver abcesses'.[42] The use of weighted preferences proceeds by seeking patient, health workers' relatives' or public preferences between different pairs of states of ill health, then statistically processing these to yield consistent weightings. Some early QALY values for different states of health were derived in this way.[43] Imputing cash values to different states of ill health can be done actuarially or by considering court awards[44] or from the actual costs of ill health to the NHS, employers, families, etc.

4 Pilot test the candidate to ascertain how far it satisfies the above criteria. Managers and marketers should be able to determine for themselves whether the proposed indicator is general or specific enough, whether it covers the relevant aspects of the service and uses available data. Clinical pertinence, the degree of certainty and face validity can be established by consultation with clinicians. Establishing precision, sensitivity and reliability requires experiments. The NHS marketer would be advised to entrust these to a clinician or other professional researcher. Many texts explain the techniques and supporting theory more fully than is possible here.[45] Internal validity will also have to be established by experiment unless relevant research has already been published.

5 Modify the candidate outcome indicator in the light of step 4 (unless the candidate outcome indicator satisfies all the above criteria first time) and repeat steps 4 and 5 until a satisfactory indicator is found. This is the most time-consuming part of the process.

Chapter 4

Market research in the NHS

Using market research as a decision support technique

The purpose of market research is to inform decisions. Hence the manager responsible for a marketing in a given NHS service should also be the manager responsible for commissioning the market research, receiving the results and for acting upon them. The previous chapter and the next two list the main decisions to which the NHS might apply market research. Essentially the same process is required for all types of NHS market research. Figure 4.1 outlines how NHS market research can be done and this section explains the main steps (labelled A to L to avoid confusion with steps in the overall marketing process described in other chapters). Steps A to F show how to decide a market research package for a DHA, unit or general practice, steps G to L show how to implement it.

NHS market research can often be completed in two or three months but in practice the main causes of delay are:

- Slowness in deriving a market research brief. A balance has to be struck between getting a precise, clear brief (see step A below) and avoiding interminable consultations.
- Over-consultation about the wording of questionnaires or other data collection instruments which consequently go through many drafts.
- Getting NHS staff who are new to market research to understand what is required and why, and building up their self-confidence to begin.
- Failing to collect comparator or control data from the outset, so that this data has then to be collected after data on one's own service instead of simultaneously.

Beside supporting marketing decisions, market research has promotional effects which have to be taken into account when managing market research. Market research is a sign of the NHS organization's willingness to consider its users' wishes. Letting respondents know what will be done with their answers and what benefits might follow reinforces this, as does publication of

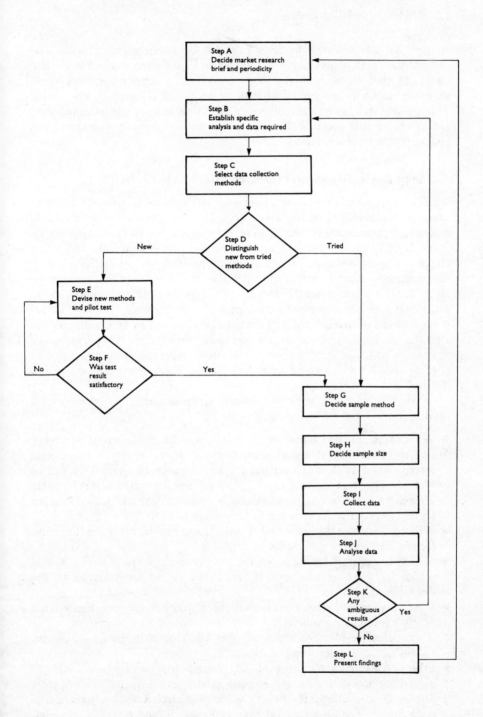

Figure 4.1 The market research cycle

results. Market research findings can also be communicated inside and outside the NHS organization to explain and legitimize action based upon them. Market research should not be used as an opportunity for salesmanship, arguably not even for health promotion. (The ethical codes of the Market Research Society and other organizations which emphasize this may reflect a belief that salesmanship would tend to discredit market research and reduce future response rates.)

Step A. Decide market research brief and periodicity

What market research analyses, data and data collection methods an NHS manager will require depends upon what decisions the market research is to inform (i.e. which stage of the NHS marketing process the market research is being conducted for). Models outlined in the previous and the following chapters suggest the types of NHS market research shown in Table 4.1. A unit's market research programme will therefore consist of whatever items from Table 4.1 are currently relevant to the unit's managerial activities. In practice it may be necessary (to save money and above all time) to conduct several pieces of market research simultaneously (e.g. to decide whether to alter the specification of a service whilst meanwhile tracking its performance against its existing specification). Then it is especially important not to confuse the different analyses and data relating to different but concurrent decisions.

The best way to clarify these points at the outset is by drawing up a market research brief which states at least:

- What decisions the market research is to inform. For instance one NHS manager suspected that staff in his department might require training in interpersonal skills and initiated market research to check this and to identify what training to provide. This requires data on how service users viewed the staff's interpersonal skills and to compare staff with user perceptions of the department.
- Who makes these decisions and when. This gives the main deadlines and feedback routes for the results.
- Which target population of 'customers' to research (see Chapter 3) and which of these groups' beliefs, behaviours, etc. are relevant to the decisions to be taken.
- What services and what aspects of them are to be researched, hence what analytic results are required.
- If statistical results are required, the tolerable margins of error and confidence levels (see step H, p. 99).
- Ethical considerations; rules of data confidentiality or permissions required for access to patients. Among others, the Association of Market Survey Organisations, the British Market Research Society and the European Society for Opinion and Market Research (and their constituents) adhere to codes of ethics in market researching.[1]

Table 4.1　Types of NHS market research

Decision	MR analysis	Data required
What services to buy (or provide through DMUs)?	Influences on referral patterns and health behaviour	Population preferences and perceptions of alternate health services. Marketing strength/weakness of non-NHS services
	How far GP referral patterns reflect population need for health services	What groups seeking care do not present to GP and why
	Segmentation by locality	Travel, working, consumption and social preferences and habits of clients and informal carers
What SGT services to sell?	SWOT, sales forecasts, market types, environmental scanning	Market sizes and shares, their determinants. Competitor performances and plans
		Buyer income and demands
		User behaviour and preferences
		Own and competitors' USPs
		Policy and technical changes
		Demographic and social setting
		GP referral patterns and their determinants (with or without practice budgets)
Setting quality specifications and service design	Quality chain	Events and key decision points in the patient episode
Provider-led elements; evaluation	Analysis of substitute/competitor services' best performance, R&D, innovations	Technologies available, their cost and effectiveness in practice, acceptability to users
	Identification of 'market' leaders in buyer or user eyes	Buyer or user perceptions and preference
	User-led outcome indicators	Users' views on outcomes
User-led elements	Specification of content – no analysis: standards 'read off' from data	User preferences, expectations experiences of services; knowledge of health services and health behaviours, attitudes to competitors and substitutes. Demands of informal carers
	Segmentation	User preferences demographic and social profile, experience of local services, living, working and consumption patterns

Table 4.1   *continued*

Decision	MR analysis	Data required
Selling services (income generation)	Market types	Prospective buyers, size of their budgets, market trends. Analysis of competing/substitute providers' USPs
	Content of services: no analysis – 'read off' from buyer preferences	Buyer preferences and what influences these. Who makes the decision to buy
Which should be core services?	Which services have to be provided locally?	Users' transport resources, living and working patterns. Knowledge of service availability, willingness to use locally-provided services
Communication strategy	Difference between users' and buyers' actual beliefs attitudes and behaviours and those necessary to realise business plan	Buyers', users' and staff beliefs, attitudes and behaviours and their determinants
	Differences between users/buyers and staff perceptions of services	Media representation of existing or proposed services
	Segmentation	Patterns in buyer and user demography, health behaviour. Social mix, epidemiology or health care intervention corresponding to difference in belief attitude or behaviour
Acceptability of new service or product	Compare effects of new service or product with those required to meet shortfalls in service specification or business plan implementation	Acceptability to users/buyers of service characteristics: acceptability to informal carers
Staff recruitment	Compare what organization is perceived to offer staff with what staff seek	Preferences of potential staff and what influences these Perception of the organization and its reward policy compared with competitors'
Tracking Buyer tracking of SGT services	Compare key aspects of service specification/ contact with provider performance	Access to provider premises, records and patients. User experience and perceptions on user-led aspects of service

Decision	MR analysis	Data required
DHA tracking of DMU services	Comparison with plan objectives or service contract	Evaluation (clinical, epidemiological, administrative) data on provider-led aspects of service GPs' audit of discharges and hospital services' outcome and appropriateness of care
FHSA tracking of GP services	Suitability of GP referrals to hospital Whether GP services match service specifications	Hospital medical audit summaries. Acceptability of services to patients, informed carers Outcome and acceptability data. Summary of GPs' medical audit
Whether to explore critical areas in depth	Compare service performance on key variables with 'trigger' level	Causes of reaching the 'trigger' level
Promotional strategy	Compare demand with external public's knowledge, attitudes and behaviour	Users', buyers', public, internal carers' and GPs' knowledge, attitudes and behaviour
Internal tracking	Compare external performance with service specification contract business plan and other internal objectives	Clinical audit summaries; outcomes and avoidable iatrogenesis. User experiences Utilization and user preferences

- Who sponsors the research, i.e. who has authority to vary the research brief and to whom the results and analysis shall be presented.
- The deadline for completion and presentation of results.

In practice deciding the market research brief is what NHS managers often find most difficult but time and trouble taken at this stage simplifies and expedites the later steps.

NHS market research has to be done periodically if much is to be gained from it. The periodicity of market research has also to be decided at the outset. It depends upon:

- The type of decisions being supported and hence the type of market research. Delivery of SGT services to contracted quantity and quality must, for instance, be assessed thoroughly at least annually and before each

contract renegotiation. Routine tracking may have to be continuous, market research for business planning biennially or less often.
- Frequency of meetings to whom the results are to be reported.
- Requirements to co-ordinate market research with other periodic activities (budgeting, health profiling, mandatory statistical returns to central government, etc.).
- How long it takes effects of changes in the service or its environment to become perceptible hence monitorable.[2] Changes in the dental health or the age–sex mix of a population may take years to become apparent but the changes resulting from staff retraining may become visible within weeks or less.

Step B. Establish specific analysis and data required

What information is needed to make rational decisions on needs, priorities and outcomes depends upon what stage of the NHS marketing process the market research is to serve. Table 4.1 also links the main types of NHS market research with the corresponding forms of analysis and data requirements. Deciding what services an NHS buyer should buy or provide through its DMUs requires health profiles, locality planning and analysis of GP referral patterns not market research as conventionally understood. Nevertheless market research methods can contribute some (not all) of the data necessary for these activities and for identifying what influences health behaviours and service uptake. Similarly evaluations used in setting the provider-led aspects of quality specifications and testing new services are not themselves market research but market research can sometimes contribute some of the data required. Table 4.1 assumes that the essence of a 'core service' is still that it must be provided locally (despite the recent changes in definition; see Chapter 5). Market research can contribute to this. In these cases the corresponding 'analysis required' entry in Table 4.1 therefore concentrates on these secondary contributions not the main planning data required. The data required for setting service specifications, for business planning and for tracking are explained more fully in the respective chapters. Analysis of the market research often demands additional data to the service data mentioned in Table 4.1. The decision of what data to collect should also consider:

- Logical relevance of the data. For instance, in managing waiting times a manager may wish to know how long patients wait. The logically relevant data is observational data or data taken from administrative booking systems not opinion survey data. The latter tells you how long patients *think* they waited – a different question to how long they actually waited.
- The possibility of cross-checking data from different sources about the same aspect of the service ('triangulation'). For example survey responses about patients' geographical distribution might be compared with the distribution suggested by a sample of administrative data. Triangulation is

a precaution against error when market research data has to be collected quickly and cheaply by comparatively crude methods.

- Control data are required for assessing causal connections between such factors as changes in service specifications and changes in user behaviour or preferences in the recipient ('experimental') group of users. Control groups have to be selected or stratified to match the experimental data as closely as possible and to be of similar size. Control data have to be collected as frequently as the experimental data. Having a control group thus doubles the quantity of data required. Various texts describe the purpose of control data in greater depth than is possible here.[3]
- 'Time series' of data are required to identify environmental trends (is the standard or service provision improving or deteriorating? is the patient mix changing?) and monitor changes in service delivery and effect.
- Data requirements for segmenting the clientele must be decided at the outset. One cannot relate 'customer' replies and behaviours to their clinical, social or other characteristics unless this data is collected simultaneously and linked 'customer' by 'customer' to their other replies.
- Data on competitor, substitute or 'good practice' providers is most usefully comparable if it covers the same period as the data on one's own services and uses the same indicators.

Step C. Select data collection methods

Many methods for collecting primary market research data on the subjects listed in Table 4.1 are available to the NHS besides the patient questionnaires on which NHS managers tend to rely. Even the following list is not exhaustive:

- Critical Incident Analysis. This is the application of open, non-leading questions to elicit from patients what aspects of their contact with the NHS they found most memorable, best and worst.[4] It is useful for discovering the 'critical points' in the quality chain.
- Psychometric techniques such as a repertory grid[5] can be used to profile the attitudes and motivation of service users with a view to seeking possible selling points and discovering any psychological segmentation. They can also be used to assess user reaction to promotional materials.
- One-to-one interviews can be structured (i.e. using standardized sets of questions) or unstructured. They can be used to explore issues which users may be unwilling to commit to paper but may discuss with a sensitive interviewer (e.g. anxieties about particular members of staff or personal needs). In the form of meetings and networking this method is particularly important for sellers researching buyers' demands and intentions in the NHS internal market.
- Focus groups consist of a group of users with a single researcher who 'focuses' by (for example) steering patients away from discussing their personal illness and showing their scars towards discussion of the issues that interest the market researcher.

- Telephone surveys are a less laborious alternative to interviews and focus groups but tend to produce a sample representative of certain types of telephone owner.
- Patient panels can consist of either a permanent membership or of a membership replaced by rota. They provide a way of sounding out patient opinion on possible new forms of service and a source of comment on changes in service provision.
- Measurement gives simple direct access to many aspects of the service such as waiting times, food or room temperatures, patterns of telephone use, or when patients are woken (from the power surge as lights and other equipment are switched on). Its main marketing uses include monitoring implementation of service specifications and operational policies.
- Observation includes ward, site or clinical rounds ('management by walking about'[6]), the use of structured observation checklists and unstructured observation by skilled observers. Its main marketing uses are in reconstructing the quality chain and in monitoring implementation of service specifications and operational policies. Video can be used to record the body language of staff and patients as a clue to their satisfactions and frustrations.
- Questionnaires can be completed by respondents themselves, on site (e.g. as comment cards) or off it (with questionnaires distributed and collected postally), or by staff using the questionnaire to structure an interview. Questionnaires which collect scores on patient satisfaction indicators provide broad, subjective data but most market research projects will also require more probing, and objective, data.
- Ghost shopping consists of getting staff or volunteers to become patients or clients having been briefed beforehand on what to observe and how, and reporting their findings afterwards. Obviously this is not practicable for all services (e.g. major surgery) but a substitute is to follow a selected patient or client through the system. These methods are most useful for reconstructing the quality chain and for monitoring as Vignette 4.1 illustrates.
- Opinion polling can be used to examine knowledge of health behaviour or health services as well attitudes or opinions. Many well-known firms sell commercial polling services.
- Public meetings, including DHA and other NHS meetings, allow detailed discussion of NHS matters with the most interested (often the best informed and the most antagonistic) members of the public. They provide a means for testing the acceptability of service changes but otherwise are of limited market research use.
- Clinical audit summaries are of use primarily for tracking the iatrogenesis and outcomes of clinical procedures, and their conformity to safety standards and to other aspects of the service specification and operational policies. Generalized summaries of the results are likely to be of greater marketing use than clinical audit results at the level of individual cases. So are the 'service audit' forms of clinical audit which scrutinize all clinical

---

Vignette 4.1   What it's really like

To assess the quality of care in its residential homes for elderly people, Norfolk Social Services arranged for 37 elderly volunteers to be admitted as residents for a week in 37 of the Council's 46 homes. The volunteers were recruited by a newspaper advertisement and paid expenses and a small fee. As far as possible, their admission arrangements imitated those of any other resident, except that staff in the homes were told in advance of the experiment. The 'ghost shoppers' experiences were recorded in diaries and in de-briefing interviews after the week's residence.

Their findings gave a rich, qualitative picture of life in the homes. The residents' welcome to the home was usually warm although some of the admission procedures showed scope for improvement. The daily routine, especially meals, was found to run earlier than the new residents were used to at home. The importance of food and mealtimes became very evident. For instance, cups of tea are valued as much as a symbol of care and (if the residents were able to make their own tea) of independence. They also value a building layout which allowed residents to form small social groups – suggesting that small modern homes and converted older houses are the optimal type of home building, provided the rooms are not too small. Data on privacy, security, choice and relations with staff emerged, as did the comparators against which residents compare elderly persons' homes: hospitals, hotels, prison or work-house or schools. The managerial lesson learnt was that enabling staff and residents to work towards extending residents' choices and influence over the services provided requires further, and more subtle, methods than a standing consultative committee.

Source: Casey, B. – *Tell Us What It's Really Like to be a Resident in Local Authority Care in Norfolk in 1988* Norwich 1989 (Norfolk CC)

---

aspects of the quality chain, rather than those results of clinical audit which focus on individual clinicians. The question of access to clinical audit results is discussed in Chapter 6 where, as a tracking method, clinical audit is discussed more fully.

- Clinical trials provide evaluative data on outcomes, iatrogenesis and safety which can assist the setting of service quality specifications and the selection of new forms of service provision.
- Study visits are a means to investigate 'good practice', contrasting the actual effects of this practice with the claims made in research publications or promotional materials.
- Newspaper cuttings services can provide summaries of newspaper coverage of an NHS service, or of health policy or health promotion issues, which can be used to track the impact of promotional activity. So can other methods of checking media coverage such as using the indexes and recent back copies of national newspapers and periodicals.
- Inspectorial visits by NHS bodies (CHC, HAS, NRT, etc.), by other statutory bodies (HASAWE, SSI, etc.) or by voluntary organizations, and

study tours, can provide expert advice on the physical environment and methods of working. Some of these bodies' inspection handbooks provide useful checklists for good practice and tracking the achievement of safety and other minimum care standards, for instance the SSI's *Homes are for Living In*.[7] Accreditation (see also Chapter 5) is of a limited use for market research because most existing forms of accreditation focus on resources and managerial systems.

- Semantic differentiation invites respondents to categorize a service in terms of verbal continua (e.g. whether they consider a certain clinic friendly or impersonal, organized or chaotic). Its main use is in identifying targets for promotional activity or for changing the presentational aspects of a service.
- Image profiling consists of reconstructing the 'image' (i.e. the totality of beliefs and impressions) users have of a given product or service. Various methods may be used (questionnaires, interviews, etc.) and the results contribute to the formulation of a communications strategy (see Chapter 5).

To these can be added a range of secondary methods ('secondary' in the sense of using data already collected for other purposes):

- 'Leading edge' expert advice provides knowledge of likely new technical developments, especially in clinical matters and health policy or legislation. It is therefore of greatest use in setting service specifications and evaluating possible new forms of service provision. At least one Health Authority (South Tees) has already applied this method to all its main acute services.
- Accreditation is, in its existing forms, a vehicle for systematic external reviews of procedures, managerial systems, physical infrastructure and resources. This sheds some light on how services compare with 'good practice' elsewhere but yields at best only proxy data on outcomes, patients' preferences, iatrogenesis, etc.
- Administrative data, both qualitative (e.g. formal complaints files, ward procedures) and quantitative (e.g. utilization data), can contribute to reconstructing the quality chain and to tracking implementation of service specifications and operational policies.
- Mapping, for instance from OPCS or local authority data or epidemiological mapping,[8] can be used to aid segmentation, the selection of core services (from the study of travel isochrones, positions of residential areas, workplaces and routes), to reconstruct the quality chain and assess projected new services.
- Pressure and interest group opinion can advise on good practice, the acceptability of new services and the most glaring failures of communication or to meet existing service specifications. NAWCH publications (and their European counterpart) on the quality of paediatric services are an instance.[9]
- Staff opinion is of value in identifying staff training needs, in recon-

structing the quality chain and monitoring implementation of service specifications and operational policies.

- Ethics committees and ethicists can advise on the ethical acceptability of new clinical procedures; the former on clinical innovations and trials, the latter on the management of 'difficult' cases in reproductive technology, transplantation and terminal care.
- Research databases provide access to descriptions and evaluations of 'good practice'. Such databases are accessible via some medical, university and polytechnic libraries, the Department of Health and the Kings Fund Centre. They can be supplemented by the traditional, library-based methods of accessing research findings.
- Commercial databases mainly record companies' financial activities and are of little use for NHS marketing purposes except the financial appraisal of commercial suppliers (see Chapter 6). A few health-industry wide commercial databases exist, but mainly for such areas as pharmaceuticals, equipment and private acute hospitals. They mainly exist to collect and sell raw data, but some will also sell data analysis and interpretation services.
- Other NHS surveys give a clue as to the issues likely to concern users of one's own services but are better used to suggest issues to research directly than as a source of currently valid data (unless the survey appears recent, technically competent and local). A few summaries and lists have been published but these are certainly incomplete.[10] Even now NHS surveys are comparatively scarce and pressures of commercial confidentiality in the internal market may make future NHS organizations reluctant to provide copies. (Commercial health services would not even entertain the idea.)
- Periodicals, especially women's magazines and consumer publications (e.g. *Which*), often print surveys of NHS services, especially general medical practice. What some lack in scientificity they often compensate for in the size of sample and in offering a fresh, outside view.
- Newscutting and the other methods of media tracking mentioned above also provide secondary data on the views of journalists, editors, etc. which may influence public opinion.
- Market research and opinion poll organizations will sometimes provide free, or sell, copies of market research data collected for other organizations. However recent commercially or politically sensitive data is rarely obtainable in this way.

Between them the above methods are applicable to data collection for all the types of market research listed in Table 4.1. The choice of data collection methods thus depends upon the decisions to be taken and hence the data required (see above). Since each method has its own advantages and disadvantages, when selecting data collection methods it is necessary to consider how to balance:

- Breadth of data and depth. Some data collection methods (e.g. opinion polling, questionnaires) collect data on a wide, representative scale but at the cost of using standardized – and perhaps leading or misfocused – questions and without any *built-in* follow-up. Others (e.g. unstructured one-to-one interviews, critical incident analysis) are difficult to apply or summarize over a wide scale but provide 'deeper' knowledge of (say) the structure of user perceptions or motives, or the social causes of changes in health behaviours.

- Objective and subjective data. Some data collection methods (e.g. measurement, observation) collect observable and behavioural data, others (e.g. questionnaires) provide only data concerning individuals' beliefs, emotions, etc. For example, data on actual ward temperature can only be collected with a thermometer, data on whether the ward felt too hot or too cold only by asking patients or staff; the method used to answer one question does not necessarily yield data that will answer the other.
- Answers to open and closed questions. When one is trying to identify buyer or user preferences and perceptions about services, to identify areas in which to develop new services or in which existing services require remedial action, more open questions and supplementary questions are required (e.g. 'Which general practice locally offers the best service to its patients? Why do you mention that practice?'). For tracking and setting user-led specifications more closed, structured questions are required (e.g. 'How much time would you expect to have with the doctor? Did the doctor tell you what would happen to you next?')
- Practicable data collection methods are desirable; different skills, time and other resources are necessary for applying the chosen methods of data collection, and the costs of different methods vary greatly. In general answers to open questions about subjective matters are less easy to summarize than answers to closed questions or objective, measurable data. Practicability is discussed at step G below.

How to combine these considerations is best illustrated by examples. Assessing local population wishes as part of business planning and service quality specification requires a mixture of largely subjective methods (questionaires, interviews) with an emphasis on breadth, and using open questions. To assess their needs requires largely objective methods (epidemiological and social profiling), again with an emphasis on breadth of data. To find GP referral patterns, especially for GPs with practice budgets, would require a combination of objective methods (e.g. administrative data on referral patterns, cross-boundary flow) to give a broad picture and subjective data, pursuing in depth (e.g. through interviews, telephone surveys) the GPs' reasons for their preferred patterns of referral. To consult GPs routinely on their monitoring of hospital services would require broad, subjective data (e.g. collected by questionnaires). Discovering GPs' preferences about the nature, costs, quality of local services might involve detailed but subjective data obtained by open questions to the LMC and other professional bodies or to meetings and focus groups, all supplemented by some broader, closed methods (e.g. opinion polling) to check the representativeness of these views. Lastly, finding out what quality issues are selling points for GPs, buyers or the public would require subjective data produced by open questioning through wide-scale methods (e.g. postal survey) supplemented by more detailed methods (e.g. critical incident analysis) to expose the interpretation of these preferences and their reasons.

Nearly all NHS market research activities therefore require not one but a combination of data collection methods. Vignette 4.2 shows the combination of methods used in one hospital department. In deciding what methods to combine it is also necessary to consider:

- Complementarity of methods. This can provide a means to interpret initial market research results. Having, for instance, discovered by questionnaire that patients find (say) the clinic environment unsatisfactory one might then wish to know what aspects they find unsatisfactory, what they are tacitly comparing the clinic with (other nearby clinics, bank or supermarket premises?) and what they would regard as the desirable environmental standards. Interviews or focus groups might be required to find this out. The questionnaire indicates how widespread these dissatisfactions are, interviews or focus groups interpret and diagnose them. Using the same method of data collection to serve several market research projects at once obviously saves time and money but one must avoid the risk of creating complex and over-long questionnaires, interviews etc.
- Duplication of methods (e.g. to collect user opinions regarding which are the best and the worst aspects of a service by both questionnaire and focus groups). This allows triangulation of the results where greater confidence is required but obviously increases the time and cost of the market research.
- Sequencing the methods. Two benefits arise from doing the secondary data collection before the primary. One may discover that the data one seeks already exist; and secondary data can provide models for data collection methods and suggest issues likely to interest users of one's own services. Primary data collection can be simplified by using one data collection method as the means to organize another, e.g. by including in a questionnaire a question asking respondents who are willing to take part in a focus group or telephone survey to give a name and phone number. The risk in doing so is to multiply bias; questionnaire respondents might not be representative of the client group, and volunteers for interview not representative of respondents.

Developing market research instruments

Step D. Distinguish new from tried methods

NHS managers sometimes take the short cut of borrowing (or borrowing and adapting) data collection instruments (e.g. questionnaires, checklists) developed by other organizations such as the Kings Fund or UMIST questionnaires. This can save the delay, costs and risks of developing and piloting one's own methods and provide comparability of data across services. Borrowing is justifiable if, but only if:

- The data produced by the instrument are actually relevant to one's own managerial decisions. It is (for instance) unlikely that data yielded by someone else's tracking instruments will match the specifications of one's own service contracts (unless the service contract has been drafted with that in mind).
- There is already evidence that the instrument has been validated and applied successfully (the criteria of 'success' are outlined below).
- The time, staff and other resources necessary to use it and to process the results are available locally.
- The data generated using the instrument elsewhere are also accessible; otherwise the advantage of comparability is lost.

It is also prudent to check whether the instruments are protected by copyright. The same considerations apply to re-using data collection methods developed in one's own organization. Revising a borrowed questionnaire may lead to the worst of both worlds; a validated instrument is lost, the costs and risks of developing a new instrument are incurred and the end product may still not be tailored very closely to local needs. Piloting may be advisable even for an instrument validated elsewhere if there is reason to believe local conditions may differ significantly from those in which validation first occurred. For data collection methods satisfying all these conditions one can omit steps E and F in Figure 4.1 and proceed directly to step G. Other methods count as 'new' for present purposes. They include familiar techniques (e.g. checklists, questionnaires) in new forms (here, with new items or questions respectively).

Step E. Devise new methods and pilot test

The process for devising new market research instruments, under any of the above headings, is essentially the same as for developing outcome indicators (see Chapter 3, pp. 73f.).

To minimize bias a data collection method must firstly maximize response. In decreasing order of effectiveness, tactics for achieving this include:

- Developing data collection methods which minimize respondent discretion to participate. On this count collecting data from a medical record is preferable to collecting it from voluntary questionnaires.
- Making voluntary data collection media 'user friendly': attractive, simple to participate in, providing acknowledgement for the respondent's contribution and above all quick to complete.
- Offering rewards for responses. One holiday firm enters the questionnaires of respondents who are willing to supply their name and address into a monthly lottery whose prize is a new car.

Vignette 4.2   Market research in an accident and emergency department

Leicester Royal Infirmary decided in 1988 to assess their Accident and Emergency Department using a market research approach. To build up a rounded picture, five data collection methods were used over a short period in the summer of 1988. To indicate issues which might concern Leicester Accident and Emergency patients, and which other data collection methods might address, a synopsis of the results of research in A &E and out-patients services elsewhere was produced by the Health Services Management Unit, Manchester University. Questionnaires were then devised for both patients and staff, the two questionnaires' questions matching wherever possible to allow for later comparison of staff with patient views. The questionnaires were distributed to and collected from A & E patients with help from Leicester CHC, and distributed to staff simultaneously. One question asked whether the respondent would be willing to take part in a telephone survey and if so to provide names and telephone numbers. A random sample of those who did were then telephoned and asked to explain and elaborate points they had made in their questionnaire answers. For instance, someone who mentioned furnishings was asked what standard the A & E waiting room should be furnished to (like a hotel? or airport lounge? a private home?). Two focus group meetings were held with staff, and a discussion with the CHC Secretary. There were very few low-quality, facetious or otherwise unusable responses to these data collection methods.

- Making contingency plans to replace respondents who drop out.
- Making contingency plans to chase up respondents who don't reply. Personally-addressed reminders can increase response rates by up to 20%.[11]
- Estimate the number of observations, records, questionnaires, etc. to allow for non-responses (see step H).
- Analyse and present the data in ways that minimize the extent to which validity of the results is sensitive to a low response rate (e.g. by not jumping to conclusions about extreme findings on small groups of respondents).

Table 4.2 illustrates how to apply other strategies for minimising bias and producing clear, valid answers in designing a questionnaire. Analogous points apply to interview schedules, observation checklists and other data collection methods. An extensive literature can give more detailed advice on these matters than space allows here.[12]

Pilot testing new data collection methods prolongs the wait for the first market research results but can obviate the waste of time and money later (see step J) by resolving any unforeseen difficulties. The pilot test simply consists of using the new method in conditions as similar as possible to those of the market research itself but on a smaller scale. Not only the collection of data must be tested but also the time and logistic requirements to process the

Table 4.2   Thirteen rules-of-thumb for questionnaire design

1   Make the questions or sets of statements for respondents to agree or disagree with as specific, succinct and clear as possible; all else being equal, 'Did ward staff give understandable replies to your questions?' is preferable to 'Were the hospital staff you met generally helpful to you and other people?' In general the more focused and specific a closed question is, the less ambiguous the responses and the more critical. Very general questions tend to yield more expressions of satisfaction.

2   Use each question to elicit only one piece of information. 'Did the doctor give you the information you wanted?' will yield a fairly unambiguous answer; 'Did doctors, nurses and paramedical staff give you the information and the time that you wanted?' will not.

3   Move from more general to more specific questions ('funnelling') not the reverse.

4   Leave personal questions (about age, occupation, etc.) until last.

5   Sequence questions so that replies to earlier questions do not bias replies to later questions.[13]

6   Check phrases and questions for ambiguity; expressions such as 'waiting time' bear many different interpretations.

7   Minimize 'filtering', i.e. routing respondents or data collectors through different sets of questions or observations according to earlier answers (e.g. 'If "yes" go to question 17B.').

8   Avoid questions requiring the respondent to give embarrassing or self-incriminatory answers (e.g. 'What do you earn?' or 'Why did you fail to reply to the hospital's letter?' respectively). Respondents will rationalize.[14]

9   Avoid leading questions e.g. 'When did the nurses wake you up?'

10   Avoid questions which will elicit conventionally polite answers e.g. 'Did our staff provide good treatment?' Respondents will tend to give the conventionally expected answer.[15]

11   Avoid very difficult or demanding questions, e.g. about trivial events which happened a long time ago.[16]

12   Minimize the number of questions: ideally ask fewer than 20.

13   Draft questions to match the general public's reading age of around nine.[17] Drafts can be checked for this by an educationalist or psychologist.

results, and whether staff will require any special training to collect or to analyse the data. The achievable response rates, and how long it takes to achieve these can also be noted. As few as ten or twenty uses of an observation checklist, questionnaire or measuring system can establish its practicability and intelligibility (see below). To establish its criterion-related validity by comparing the results given by the new method with those given by other indicators will require a pilot on a similar scale to the market research itself (see step G).

Step F. Check whether the new method was satisfactory in pilot tests

The new method can be judged satisfactory insofar as the instrument:

- Gives a valid indication of the data required; the different senses of 'validity' and how they are tested are outlined in the previous section and in the various texts on research methods[18] and market research.[19]
- Yields the data required, concisely and unambiguously. This may require supplementary explanations or definitions of questions for the user (e.g. 'Take "Doctor" to mean "family doctor", "school doctor" or "hospital doctor".')
- Generates, in the case of broad data collection methods, an adequate response rate. In practice NHS questionnaires usually generate response rates in the range 30–70% of eligible respondents; a target in the upper half of this range should generally be achievable.[20]
- Spreads the responses. A multi-choice question or observation check which places most responses or observations in just one category should be redrafted with this category sub-divided to increase the spread and discrimination of results.
- Has instructions for use that are comprehensible to its users and these do in practice collect the data intended.
- Is practicable to use. For instance, if a single observer is to use an observation checklist, does the site layout allow one person to make all the required observations in the right order and fast enough? Is it possible to record all the data in the form and space provided?
- Is intelligible and acceptable to the respondents. Large numbers of non-responses or 'don't knows' may indicate a badly-drafted questionnaire or checklist. One finely-typed questionnaire in a Yorkshire hospital got a low response; enquiries revealed that it had been distributed in the ophthalmology clinic.
- Yields data that are processible given the staff, time and information systems available, and processible on the full-scale of market research anticipated. To check the latter simply multiply the time taken to process each form, interview, phone call (or whatever) by the desired number of responses to find the commitment of staff time alone.
- Is acceptable to staff in the services under scrutiny.

If the instrument proves unsatisfactory on any of these points it may be necessary to supplement the pilot test with further interviews with users and respondents to try to identify causes of the main faults. Once the instrument has been adapted accordingly, step E and this step can be repeated.

Carrying out the market research

Step G. Decide sampling method

Care in the choice of sampling method is more necessary when one seeks broad, representative data and less critical (and is a choice from different methods than those outlined below) when seeking deep, interpretative data rather than broad, representative data. When seeking interpretative data sample sizes can for practical NHS marketing processes be small; 50 (or even fewer) interviews or telephone conversations suffice for most purposes. In either case the more far-reaching the consequences of the decision are likely to be, the greater the confidence required in the market research results and the greater the quantity and types of data it will be prudent to collect. The main practicable sampling methods for seeking representative data are listed below, in decreasing order of likelihood that they will produce an unbiased sample:

- Probability sampling, in which every member of the target population stands an equal chance of being interviewed, observed, given a question-naire or whatever, and the total size of the population is known. Prob-ability sampling can therefore be applied to exhaustive lists of data such as general practice or discharge lists. Computerized information systems can easily generate probability samples from such lists. Probability sampling is preferable if statistical processing of the results is intended. However neither probability nor random sampling of a large target population is a cost-effective way to ensure data represents small minority sub-populations.
- Random sampling, differing from probability sampling in that the total population size is unknown, restricting the scope for statistical processing. It too can readily be done using computerized patient information systems.
- Systematic sampling (also called 'file sampling') chooses the first respon-dent randomly from a list and then samples every 'nth' name thereafter. This is also easy to do from a computerized patient information system but can only be applied to homogeneous 'customer' groups (e.g. users of a health screening or post-treatment review programmes).
- Cluster sampling divides the target population into representative clusters then samples one at random. For NHS work, data collection is often easier on a 'cluster' basis, taking (for instance) a non-bank holiday week's throughput of patients or a locality as the cluster.
- Stratified random sampling divides the target population into strata, applies random sampling within each stratum, and then weights any results by the size of each stratum to produce statistics about the whole population. This enables the marketer to take a systematic view of all the 'customer' segments, especially minorities such as sufferers from rare conditions or diseases, but is only practicable if the marketer already has secondary market research data to indicate which differences within the target population (e.g. of age, sex, specialty) are likely to differentiate their attitudes, behaviour, or whatever else the marketer is researching.
- Quota sampling also divides the population according to the differences within the target population which are likely to differentiate their atti-tudes, behaviour, or whatever else the marketer is researching. A quota of

each sub-population are then sampled, the size of each quota reflecting how large a proportion of the whole population each sub-population is. In practice the data collector has to judge which quota a respondent belongs to. Quota sampling is widely used in non-NHS market research but for accurate results it relies heavily on the skills of the data collectors.

- Convenience (or 'accidental') sampling simply takes the required number of observations, questionnaires, etc. as accessible or convenient. This makes for quick and cheap sampling but obviously at greater risk that the sample is unrepresentative in some important respect (e.g. orthopaedics patients may be heavily over-represented in a Tuesday clinic).

Lists of possible respondents from which to sample include:

- Internal NHS sources: PAS, practice lists, master patient indexes, medical records and other administrative lists; but these only list existing and previous patients.
- Electoral registers. These are the most comprehensive publicly available lists and updated annually but even these under-record multiple occupancies, short-term occupants and non-voters (e.g. recent immigrants, children, many mentally-disordered people).
- Some specialist firms sell mailing lists, others will mail questionnaires (etc.) to respondents selected randomly or by specific criteria. These lists will have been prepared for commercial purposes and, depending on the sources, may under-record low-income groups, people who do not use credit, etc. The efficiency of these mailings should be checked by another method in view of the difficulties reported during some recent share issues.
- Market research firms will construct samples and collect data to order.
- Voluntary bodies may sometimes be willing to assist in selecting samples (and distributing questionnaires, etc.). This is of greatest use in stratified, quota and convenience sampling.

Step H. Decide sample size

In deciding how large a sample to take there are two main considerations – what size of sample is representative of the target population; and what size of sample is practically manageable. The following guidelines on sample size apply to selecting a sample of the target population. If comparisons are to be made with a control group, a sample of similar size, sampled by the same method, is required for that too.

For collecting broad, representative, quantitative data for statistical analysis the requisite sample size is one that reduces the margin of error and the probability of its being exceeded to tolerable levels. A standard formulae connects sample size, margin of error and the risk of error as follows:

$$n = \frac{s^2 . Z^2}{E_2}$$

where n is the minimum necessary sample size, s is the standard deviation in the sample and E is the margin of error acceptable in the final estimate – Gallup accept a margin of error up to $\pm 3\%$ on a 1000-person sample.[21]

Z the number of standard deviations of a sample corresponding to a given probability that statistics calculated for the sample lies within E from the real parameter in the population. (For a normally distributed population Z can be looked up in a statistical table.) How high this probability of error may be is, in most circumstances, an arbitrary choice. Usually a small, round figure is chosen such as 0.05 (5% – perhaps the most common), 0.01 (1%), or 0.001 (one in a thousand).

Different formulae are required for qualitative data and for non-normal distributions. Detailed explanations of how to estimate standard deviation in a sample, of how the formulae available for determining sample size and of how to use them are available in the many textbooks.[22]

For example, one can use the above formula to estimate what sample size has a 95% probability of yielding a figure for mean waiting time to an accuracy of plus or minus five minutes when the standard deviation for a sample of individual patients' waiting times is known to be 35 minutes. A 95% probability requires $Z = 2.0$ (approximately). Substituting in the above equation gives

$$n = 35^2 . 2^1/5^2 = 1225.4/25$$

Hence a sample of at least 196 waiting times is necessary (irrespective of how many patients there are altogether).

Rules of thumb for sample size, which may be good enough for deciding sample sizes for comparatively routine, small-scale decisions are:

- Sample sizes of greater than 200 will not often be necessary, at least for exploratory, first-time market research. For a given margin of error (E in the above equation) the probability that a given sample result lies outside this margin declines very slowly (as sample size grows) once sample size exceeds 200. Increasing sample size, and consequently costs, not so much reduces the margin of error as reduces the probability of that error, or a larger error, occurring.[23]
- In many statistical calculations the risk of error grows rapidly once sample size falls below 30, so the smallest segment which it is intended to analyse independently should not be smaller than this.
- One may analyse incoming data as it arrives and simply continue collecting data until no new gross trends are obvious (the crudest method of all).
- The total sample size must be large enough for the smallest segment or other sub-population which the researcher wishes to analyse independently still to be large enough to yield usable results.
- Add to the above a compensation for prospective respondents who drop out or fail to respond (see step E).

When market research results are challenged it is often with claims that the sample size makes the data unrepresentative. However a larger sample is not necessarily more representative than a smaller. A small (e.g. 10%) sample may be representative if there is no reason to think that the rest of the population differs from it in characteristics likely to influence their opinions or behaviours (e.g. if one is sampling a socially homogenous group on non-controversial subjects). A 10% probablistic sample may yield more accurate, less risky results than a 20% convenience sample. Strategies to improve response rates are discussed above (see steps D, E. and F).

In deciding whether a given sample size and method of sampling is practicable it is necessary to consider:

- The time required to select the sample, collect and process the data, which can be checked in a pilot test (see step E). This time must be less than the periodicity of the market research (see Step A).
- The cost of collecting the data (see next section).
- Whether sufficient staff and information systems are available for processing the data (see next section).
- Whether the data are accessible. Use of some data will be limited by requirements of medical or commercial confidentiality (e.g. psychiatric admissions lists, complaints data respectively). Other data may have to be anonymized (perhaps in regard to staff besides patients' identities) before market researchers may see it.
- Whether NHS staff, volunteers or respondents (through self-reporting are able to collect the data, and if not whether researchers, commercial market researchers or consultants can be recruited to do so. Availability of NHS staff or volunteers depends upon whether any preparatory training is necessary and can be provided (see below).

Step I. Collect data

Four further decisions have to be made before data can be collected.

- When to collect data depends on the type of market research. Data on non-users or prospective users obviously has to be collected before the start of any new NHS episode, data on buyers before negotiations on service contracts begin. Data on the quality chain and tracking data have to be collected after the care episode and around the critical points during it. Data on user experiences and longer-term outcome or iatrogenesis must be collected after the acute episode. Lastly data collection has to be completed in time for processing and analysis before the decisions it supports are to be taken.
- Where to collect data depends upon the choice of target population (including any control group) and from sampling requirements. Data on users of other services, prospective users and dischargees will probably have to be collected off site. The choice of place to collect data can assist (or obstruct) sampling; a random sample of local residents is more likely to be achieved in a shopping centre on a Saturday than at the gates of a

specialized plastics factory, but the reverse may reply if a quota of (say) manual workers aged 20–40 and exposed to carcinogens is required.

- Who is to collect the data is discussed in the next section. The main decision is whether to use the NHS organization's own staff, researchers, volunteers, the respondents' own help or a commercial market researcher. Data collectors who work in public places or door-to-door will require some form of identification or introduction document.
- Whether the data collectors are to be identified to respondents as representatives of the NHS organization. This will tend to improve response rates by taking advantage of the public popularity of the NHS and reassuring respondents that the 'market research' is not a preliminary to some kind of pressure selling. The disadvantage is that obliging respondents are likelier to soften their replies if they perceive the data collector as an NHS employee. It is considered unethical to use market research as a vehicle for selling but it is less clear whether this proscription would also extend to health promotion activities.

On the basis of these decisions one can arrange the logistics of data collection (who will distribute and collect questionnaires and other documents? what travel and access arrangements have to be made for data collectors?) Record progress in data collection so that any contingent difficulties or unexpected bias can be detected and addressed early on. Collecting data by the methods listed at step C demands:

- Interactive skills for interactive methods (interviews, focus groups, critical incident analyses, telephone surveys, panels, public meetings or study visits are to be used, or staff consulted). Essentials include use of seeking behaviours (asking for views and recommendations) not leading questions, and responding non-judgementally (not betraying surprise, disapproval, pleasure etc. explicitly or non-verbally). Open questions have often to be followed up with questions to probe answers (e.g. 'Why do you say that?' 'Compared with what?') to yield data of use to the NHS marketer. Strict conformity to questionnaire wording and sequence is necessary if structured methods are used. It is desirable to explain to respondents why their views are important to the NHS, what uses the data will be put to, and the procedure that will now be followed. It is desirable to acknowledge the respondent's help, answer any remaining questions he or she may have, and give any necessary reassurance on the confidentiality of answers.
- Observational skills for methods such as study tours, inspections, observation, measurement. Here the main skill required is to brief data collectors at the outset what data one is seeking and to try to ensure that these methods are used discreetly enough to minimize (one of) the 'Hawthorne effects': the effect that observation itself may have in changing the behaviours or attitudes of those observed.[24] In quota sampling the data collector must often be able to judge from appearances or from indirect hints or replies what social group a respondent belongs to; for sex this is

usually easy enough but not always easy for age, social class, ethnicity or degree of disability.

- Technical training in psychometrically-based methods (critical incident analysis, repertory grid, semantic and image profiling) on the application, scoring and interpretation of the instruments used. This form of data collection may have to be sub-contracted to experts or specialist firms.
- Evaluative methods (clinical audit, clinical trials, ethics committees) require knowledge both of the methods and limitations of clinical research, and a broad substantive knowledge of the state of clinical practice in the areas concerned. To take full advantage of these methods it will be necessary to involve clinicians (and perhaps ethicists) in collecting and interpreting information, but this may anyway be desirable for other reasons (see Chapter 6).
- Secondary methods (leading edge advice, reviewing other surveys, databases, periodicals, cuttings services, mapping, use of administrative data) require both knowledge of sources and the researcher's skills in tracing, collecting, summarizing, interpreting and criticizing a large mass of mainly printed data from diverse sources. Knowledge of the use of library and database systems is necessary here.

Before collecting the data, it is necessary to ensure that the data collectors have, or can be trained in, these knowledges and skills.

Step J. Analyse data

How to assess the consumers' responses, and how to analyse them, depends upon the decisions to be made using the market research results. These are outlined in discussions of the different steps in the marketing process (Chapters 3, 5 and 6) and in Table 4.1. At the outset one can check the user-friendliness of the market research. One can also note the quality of responses but before making any further analyses, one must weed out and note incomplete, misunderstood, facetious and other unusable replies. In nearly all the applications mentioned in Table 4.1 several of the following types of analyses will be required:

- Comparison with a normative benchmark. Market research results are almost uniformative unless compared with a normative benchmark and may be seriously misleading – '80% of orthopaedic patients found the doctor's explanations helpful' may induce false confidence until it is compared with a figure of 85% for three months ago and 95% for the neighbouring SGT. The benchmark may be past performance, competitors' performance, patient or public preferences, NHS policy, a control group, 'good practice', or the NHS organization's own business plan objectives, quality specification or communications strategy, as circumstances require. Figure 4.2 gives an anonymized excerpt from the analysis of market research data collected for one US teaching hospital. It is not necessary to accept 'customer' responses uncritically when making a business plan or specifying quality. If their responses differ from the normative benchmark (as is to be expected in matters of, say, health promotion) it is always open to the NHS organization to use its communication strategy to try to alter 'customer' beliefs or behaviours (see Chapter 5). Only in respect of the user-led aspects of a service specification (see Chapter 3) are 'customer' responses taken as they stand as a norm for service planning.

- Projections and time series. Commercial projections (of sales, cash turnover, activity, etc.) are especially important for business planning in SCTs, and real projections of demographic and epidemiological data for health profiling and locality planning. Hospital DMUs will need projections of GP referral patterns for their planning. Time series are necessary for tracking. Regression analysis is the standard statistical technique (but note that like all the statistical techniques it shows correlation not causation and requires qualitative interpretation too). Vignette 4.3 gives a US example of the sorts of uses projections can be put to in negotiating service contracts.
- Causal, evaluative interpretations of trends in two or more sets of data, for instance to assess the likelihood that a change in the age-mix of a resident population is connected with a change in the pattern of uptake of outpatient services and the size of any such influence. 'Significance testing' assesses how probable it is that differences between the result and the comparitor are larger than might occur by chance because samples are being compared not whole populations. This requires analysis of correlation and partial correlation by statistical techniques, then interpretation of the results to indicate whether there is a causal relation at work too, and if so what type of causal relation. DRGs and other classification systems can be used to standardize for differences in case mix or disease prevalence. These are tasks for someone with statistical training. (See also the large literature on evaluation and statistics.) Note that comparisons between groups only shed light on factors that differ between them; comparing groups in the same environment may (for instance) reveal the genetic differences between them but will conceal the effects of environmental differences of the factors being investigated.[25]
- Descriptive, 'illuminative' interpretation of qualitative data is of use in reconstructing the quality chain (see previous chapter) and in understanding the subjective aspects of user experiences of health care, for instance to answer such questions as; 'What is it about dentistry that frightens so many people off? What aspects of going to the dentist tend to heighten the anxiety and what aspects relieve it?'
- Segmentation of buyers and users can be revealed by considering both statistical correlations between data sets and descriptive interpretations of qualitative data. In theory there is no limit to the ways in which a user population might segment e.g. geographically, by transport method, social mix, ethnically, by marital status, by GP, etc. so to detect segmentation may require imagination and insight besides the ability to process data.

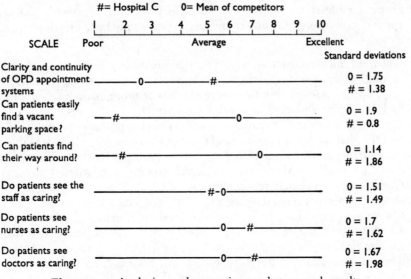

Figure 4.2 Analysing and presenting market research results

- For data generated through sampling it is prudent to analyse how probable it is that the results reflect the target populations (a common query from doctors confronted with market research findings). Besides the substantive results a statistician should be able to calculate the margin of error ('one standard error') and the probability (the 'confidence level') that the results truly represent the corresponding figure for the target population. The more far-reaching the decisions to be made on the basis of market research, the higher the confidence level that is desirable. Triangulation – comparing data on the same subject collected by different methods or from different sources – gives one check on how confidently the results can be taken. One can also check data summaries from samples against the corresponding summaries from aggregate patient or population records.[26]

All these results will often have to be combined with summaries of clinical research and evaluations, in the ways indicated in preceding and following chapters, and with the results of any secondary research which (ideally) preceded the primary market research. The analyst should also check for any contradictory or ambiguous evidence. Lastly resist the temptation to over-analyse; do the minimum analysis necessary to yield the desired information because each stage of data processing and analysis creates another opportunity for error and misinterpretation (besides increasing delays and costs). Coding qualitative answers, weighting answers to Likert or other verbal scales, combining answers to several questions and like procedures each make the results depend to a higher degree on arbitrary assumptions or weights besides the data themselves.

Step K. Are any results ambiguous?

Vignette 4.4 illustrates the sorts of ambiguity which may arise in market research data. Ambiguous market research results may have one or more of five causes:

- Apparent inconsistencies may reflect a previously unrecognized segmentation among respondents. It is not that there is no pattern to respondents' answers but that there are two or more distinct sub-groups each of which exhibits clear but different trends.
- Seemingly 'irrational' 'customer' answers or behaviour may simply reveal that the analyst doesn't understand the users' rationality.[27] In any of these cases further market research may be necessary to resolve the ambiguity. If so there is feedback in the market research process as shown in figure 4.1.
- Confused evidence may reflect a process of rapid change in the population studied, especially if the data has been collected over a long period.
- Questions or instructions in data collection instruments may have been ambiguous or the respondents more intellectually sophisticated than the questionnaire writer.[28]
- The available data may be faulty: misrecorded or miscalculated.

If any important results do appear to be ambiguous, steps B to J must be repeated with new analyses and data collection methods to disambiguate the market research.

Vignette 4.3   An American service contract negotiation

An American hospital was approached by a state agency who offered the hospital an exclusive contract to treat certain categories of publicly-funded patients. The offer stipulated in detail the fixed-rate reimbursement per case, with cases grouped by major disease category (corresponding to groups of DRGs). This is a common US practice. If the hospital's actual costs for a case exceeded the agreed reimbursement, the hospital would bear the loss or, in the reverse case, keep the profit. The hospital used a decision support system provided by a commercial software supplier to project the expected volume of cases and the expected case costs for each major disease category, and to compare the result with the total reimbursement for that number of patients. Totalled, the resulting projections for profit and cost showed that the hospital would lose heavily on the contract. However, the analysis also showed that the loss came entirely from two categories of patient, the newborn and those with circulatory diseases. Costs for these categories were then analysed by four ill-health severity levels. The analysis showed that the projected losses within these categories would result from the variable costs of treating patients with stage 3 and especially stage 4 severity. The hospital, therefore, negotiated to alter the contract reimbursement for stage 3 and 4 newborns and circulatory disease patients. This made the contract profitable and the hospital accepted it.

Source: Sales presentation, SDS PLC.

Step L. Present results

Market research findings can most usefully be presented in dual form. An 'executive summary' presents the practical, managerial implications of the findings. It should be presented in as brief and as clear a form as possible (e.g. using graphs and graphics where possible) but providing references and back-up data to substantiate any controversial or surprising conclusions and to support decisions of major importance. It draws upon the full report. This should state, probably in the following order:

- Remit of the market research.
- The target population, its size and any sampling method, stating when and where the samples were taken.
- The data that were collected.
- Assumptions and any statistical methods used when analysing them.[29]
- Results of the analyses.
- How much reliance can be placed upon the results. The report should note any possible causes of bias such as groups (e.g. patients too ill to answer) omitted from data collection.
- Which data are ambiguous and what further research would be required to resolve the ambiguities.
- Practical implications and managerial options, with the advantages and disadvantages of each.
- Any recommendations and the reasons for them.

Recommendations, and the reasons for them, should be separated from statements of facts, as should matters of conjecture or opinion. Service strengths and weakness should be given as near equal weight as the facts allow. A report which simply summarizes defects in the service is likely to be as one-sided as one which suggests everything requires little or no change. It is necessary to avoid any spurious suggestion of quantified accuracy or scientificity when the data or methods will not bear this interpretation. It may be useful to suggest experts to whom the report can be presented for a second opinion. Vignette 4.4 gives the main headings and a flavour of the content of one NHS market research report.

The results can then be presented to:

- The line manager responsible for the service researched into and who commissioned the market research. It is for the line manager to decide on the basis of this presentation what marketing strategy to adopt, including how to reconcile the conclusions of the above analysis with the other objectives of the service.
- Other managers with an interest in the service (e.g. those who receive patients referred from this service, or whose patients may be referred to it, business planners, accountants).
- Clinicians in the service concerned.
- Staff who contributed data or who will be involved in implementing the recommended action. In this way market research can be used to convince

---

Vignette 4.4 Assessing an accident and emergency service

Questionnaires, telephone surveys, meetings and secondary research were used to collect market research data on Accident and Emergency Services at the Leicester Royal Infirmary in the summer of 1988. The resulting data had then to be analysed and presented to A & E managers as a basis for their decisions about whether or how to alter A & E services and refurbish the A & E department. The report headings (in original order) were:

Managerial objectives – Decisions to be taken using the market research, including possible staff training.
Managerial findings – Summary
Service strengths – The seven main strengths were outlined; unexpectedly, they included speed of service at certain times of day.
Service deficiences – There were seven of these, one of which related to a contracted support service.
Ambiguous findings – Indicating where no clear views emerge and where further market research might be necessary.
Comparison of staff and Patient Perceptions – This was as a basis for advice on whether a training programme was indicated and, if so, of what kind.
Recommendations – Five issues requiring a management decision.

Appendices on questionnaire scores, market research methods and detailed verbatim feedback.
   The report was so drafted that it could be circulated to staff if desired. This meant that some of the patients' more pointed comments could not be quoted directly in case individual members of staff were recognizable.

---

staff, in a fairly objective way, that there really is a problem with how services are provided. In the latter two cases the presentation of unpalatable results obviously has to be both tactful and objective.

- The buyer, in the case of any seller's information (e.g. tracking information) demanded by the service contract.
- Any external bodies which have a claim to the results (e.g. the CHC, inspectorates or accreditors).
- The public or mass media, if this will advance the communications strategy (see Chapter 5). For SGTs this has to be set against the requirement for commercial confidentiality of information whose publication might aid competitors.

The market research infrastructure

Establishing a market research capability

To establish a permanent dialogue with the consumers of NHS services requires a permanent market research infrastructure (as part of a marketing function; see Chapter 6) in NHS organizations. It comprises of the staff, budgets, information systems noted below. If the line managers must, as explained previously (Chapter 4, p. 80), take responsibility for commissioning the market research, receiving and acting upon the results for their services it is critical to organize the market research infrastructure so that they can brief it to do market research on demand. The market research function treats the line managers as its 'internal customer' even if marketing or market research is represented independently at unit, SGT or HA board or directorate level. In practice much of the work of this infrastructure will consist of tracking, including supporting clinical audit (see Chapter 6).

An NHS organization's market research staff would be:

- Specialist NHS market researchers, to design market research programmes and their data collection methods, organize data collection, analyse and present the results, and take the statistical decisions associated with all this. They will require advice from clinicians where clinical evaluations are to be combined with the market research data. There is much to be said for involving clinical directors, directors of public health, general practitioners and clinical researchers (as relevant) in the market research infrastructure.
- Data collectors, who may have to be technically trained if the more complex data collection methods are used (e.g. psychometry). However, many methods can be used by clerical or medical records staff (e.g. for observation checklists, measuring, collecting administrative data). Using staff directly involved in the care of a patient group to collect market research data from their current patients is unlikely to yield valid data and is ethically questionable.
- Administrative or clerical staff will also be required to collate and record the results.
- Training and development support. This serves two purposes. First is to update staff on the state of the MR art, not only by providing the usual courses, conferences, etc. but by encouraging links with wider marketing organizations such as the Marketing Society. Secondly in the NHS of the early 1990s much development and training will probably be necessary for staff to fulfil the above roles; Chapter 6 deals with this. Training and development activity would normally require a mix of in-house activity and bought-in support from the education centres and other agencies.

Which other managerial functions it is most necessary to co-ordinate the market research infrastructure with, depends upon the NHS organization's prime objectives, in turn determined by its place in the internal market. Since SGTs' prime objectives are commercial, its market researchers will require close co-ordination with its finance function. In general practice market research would become a task for practice managers, in buying organizations a task associated with the planners, epidemiologists and Directorate of Public Health. In the directly-managed units the obvious niche, if not a role answering directly to the UGM, is with a medical directorate or medical records function. In each case the market research infrastructure is best included in the wider marketing and quality assurance infrastructure (see Chapter 6).

In deciding what information systems would be required to support the market research infrastructure it is necessary to consider:

- How to provide access to clinical information: clinical audit summaries (see Chapter 6), results of clinical evaluations and trials, and access to patient record systems as a source for data on outcomes, iatrogenesis and utilization.
- Whether to use machine readable questionnaires or other market research data collection documents (e.g. the system developed by CASPE in Bloomsbury).[30] This is likely to be labour saving if large quantities of standardized data collection documents are used but not otherwise, and may be counter-productive if it tempts NHS market researchers to force all their questions into patterns which give only machine-readable answers.
- Whether to computerize the analysis and processing of market research data. Computerized systems save labour in processing large amounts of broad, representative data from standard data collection, in producing sample lists, statistical data and projections, and in modelling. They are very much less useful in handling qualitative data. Computerized systems in NHS marketing should also be chosen for their ability to access Medline and other computerized databases.
- How to access to PAS, PIs, Korner, RMI, budgetary and other administrative systems and how these should be extended or modified for marketing purposes. The latter is often easier said than done; PAS systems are often decided on a regional or multi-regional level, making even simple modifications (e.g. to record when patients left the OPD as well as when they arrived) laborious to implement.
- How to ensure medical, and in SGTs the commercial, confidentiality of information. In respect of patient data this can be achieved by designing marketing information systems to draw off only aggregated data or anonymized data. Data Protection Act requirements must also be satisfied if a computerized marketing information system stores data on identifiable persons.

All this requires a market research budget. For small or once-off marketing projects NHS staff costs are usually hidden in another budget but this is not practicable if a permanent market research establishment is required. A realistic market research budget will be large and recurrent. Experienced market researchers will have largely to be attracted from outside the NHS and will demand commercially-comparable salaries (£20 000 and upwards). Costs of existing types of NHS staff can be calculated from pay scales in the usual way. External consultancy (see below) costs in the range £200 to £1200 per person/day at 1990 prices. How many days are required will depend on the scale and complexity of the work but for a middle-sized OPD something in the order of 5–15 days might be required. For opinion polls carried out by reputable firms expect to pay in the order of £1000 plus a fee per question (often in the range £100–£300) for a 1000-person sample. These costs may be reduced if it is possible for the firm to tag your questions onto a survey being conducted for another purpose.

Buying in market research

Until the infrastructure exists external market research services may have to be bought in either to fill gaps in expertise (e.g. in inventing a communications strategy), or to cope with simple overload of market research work, or to provide a fresh and comparatively impartial review of current services. Respondents may answer more frankly to a researcher who seems not to be directly connected with the NHS. Buying in market research raises further practical questions:

- Where to look for an external market researcher? Organizations such as the Market Research Society can provide lists of commercial marketers and some confidence that the market researchers listed are comparatively ethical and competent. Academic researchers and non-commercial health organizations include bodies such as the King Edward Hospital Fund for London, the Nuffield Provincial Hospitals Trust and the Office of Health Economics, the Royal Colleges and other professional bodies.
- What to look for in an external market researcher? Experience in commercial market research is not scarce but external researchers experienced in NHS market research are. At the time of writing (late 1990) there are probably fewer than 50 in the whole UK but if available these are preferable because the NHS still differs from other managements in important ways (e.g. the role of the medical establishment, the nature of the service offered). Academic researchers tend to work to a high standard, comparatively cheaply, and usually for mainly non-financial motives but not all understand the managerial and organizational applications and contexts of the research, nor its commercial uses.
- How to brief an external market researcher? A similar brief content is required for an external as for an internal market researcher (see step A p. 82) but payment and control details must be added. The brief for an external market research must also stipulate the price for the work, who meets incidental expenses and on what scale, rights of copyright and resale of the information, and which aspects of the work are the responsibility of the contractor and which of the NHS organization.
- How to control an external market researcher? The requirements are much the same as for controlling any contractor: a precise, explicit brief, regular meetings to discuss progress, deadlines, and provision for withholding at least part of the payment until satisfactory results are presented.
- How to use the results of an external market researcher? The results are used much as internally-produced results are; see steps A, B, and L above and the steps in Figures 3.1 and 5.1 (see Chapters 3, 5 and 6) corresponding to the entries in Table 4.1. The main difference in using results from an external source is in their credibility and legitimation; these results can usually be represented as being comparatively free from the taint of internal NHS interests or politics.

Chapter 5

NHS marketing mix

Product mix decisions: core services and service contracts

Putting an NHS business plan and a service quality specification into practice requires a set of decisions and activities which together comprise the NHS 'marketing mix'. These are often summarized as decisions on product (or in the NHS case, service), promotion, price and place; and the corresponding activities.[1] Cash pricing and costing will remain, in the short term, an ancillary issue for NHS marketing if the Department of Health succeeds in making quality rather than cost the main locus of service contracting.[2] In real terms the 'price' of the service to the user is the compliance, inconvenience, etc. demanded from them. This has been mentioned in describing the quality chain (Chapter 3) and will be encountered again as an aspect of service design (Chapter 6). The main decision on 'place' in the NHS concerns the designation of services as 'core' or 'non-core' (or 'designated' or 'non-designated'). NHS promotions are dealt with on pp. 124f. Product decisions taken are taken at four points in NHS marketing: business plan stage and quality specification stages (pp. 46f.), in selecting providers and through service design (pp. 143f.). At the business plan stage decisions are made about which products to buy or provide, much as in commercial business planning. The NHS internal market differs by adding a distinct stage of product mix decision about which to make core and non-core services, a decision required of buyers by central policy and not taken in light of NHS organizations' individual business plans.

Step 12. Is organization a buyer, seller or a DMU?

By now this question is mentioned only for the sake of logical clarity, to differentiate the roles which the various NHS organizations have in service contracting. It can be treated as a purely factual demarcation on the lines noted at step 4, where senses in which it might instead be taken as a decision point were also noted. For RHAs and DHAs the next stage in the marketing process in step 13A. For GPs with practice budgets step 13A is pre-empted by the DHA and their next step is step 14. Sellers omit steps 13A and 14 and move directly from step 13B to step 15. Marketing in directly managed units and general practices omits steps 13, 14 and 15 and resumes at step 16, except in regard to any marginal income generating activities which are examined at step 13B (as a variant of the types of selling involved in securing a service contract). See Figure 5.1.

Step 13A. Decide core services

The step is peculiar to the NHS internal market. The first problem here is to clarify what count as 'core' or 'designated' services. *Working for Patients* defines 'core' services by giving a list of specialties.[3] However a new definition of core services has emerged from at least one of the 1989 Regional Reviews, taking as 'core' services those which:

- must be provided locally (e.g. because speed of response is necessary, as with ambulances, A&E);
- have in local circumstances only one possible provider, and;
- this provider is an SGT.

Core status can be given retrospectively in face of SGT plans to change service mix or relocate services.[4]

Either way, the purpose of designating a service as 'core' is to constrain sellers to provide the service locally. This restriction still seems intended to cover public health, community-based services and other hospital services which need to be provided on a local basis, either as a matter of policy – for example, services for elderly or mentally-ill people – or on grounds of practicability – for example, district nursing and health visiting.'[5] Non-core services include those catering for less urgent conditions which allow time for patients and GPs to choose the place of care, for patients to travel (e.g. cold surgery) and for patients who wish to choose location e.g. some elderly long-stay.[6] Services not provided in every District (e.g. Regional and sub-Regional specialties) also count as non-core services. Designating services as core or non-core is therefore a decision to be made in the light of market research (see Chapter 4 and Table 3.5). Table 5.1 illustrates one way this market research might be attempted.

When the analysis of the market research results identify a service which for practical reasons must be provided locally the service contract must stipulate where the service is to be provided and that it is (or is liable to be) categorized as a 'core' service. The supporting quality specification must include the corresponding standards for access.

Step 13B. Selling

For sellers in the NHS internal market, as in other commercial settings, the prime form of 'promotion' is salesmanship. 'Selling' in the metaphorical

Table 5.1 Identifying core and non-core services through market research; an imaginary worked example

Market research brief
> To discover what services must be provided locally and why.
> To present findings to the DHA planning groups before the next DHA meeting.
> Target populations; residents, patients, GPs. etc. . . . (see Step A, p. 82).

Analyses required
> Over which aspects of services do patients and GPs necessarily exercise choice and over which aspects would they wish to exercise choice?
> For each service do patients and GPs wish to exercise choice of location?
> Importance of location, compared with other service characteristics, as criterion for choice of which health services to use.
> Segmentation within the target populations on the above questions.
> What clinical and access considerations constrain the siting of services?
> What services are required by patients and GPs in the District but on too small a scale to be practical or economic to provide locally?

Data required
(i) Objective data (from both primary and secondary research):
> Locations of health facilities in DHA and nearby, availability of providers outside the DHA, their relation to main transport routes.
> Travel isochrones for NHS facilities in the DHA and other nearby providers, for NHS transport, public transport and private transport (from ambulance services, RHAs, Department of Employment).
> Car ownership patterns geographically (OPCS) and likely changes over period of the contract.
> Mapping of age/sex/family pattern mix geographically and likely changes over the period of the contract.
> Aspects of service likely to matter to service user (from MR elsewhere; as clue to what data to collect on local preferences).
> Existing national or local standards for access times (from professional bodies, *Health Notices* and *Health Circulars*).
> Existing referral patterns and utilization patterns especially cross-boundary flow and uptake of non-NHS services.
> Points at which choices about location to refer to already exist or are already made in the quality chain.
> Technical interdependencies of existing NHS services (e.g. can clinics be resited away from laboratories?).

(ii) Target populations' views (primary research) on:
> Acceptable travel times and methods.
> Perceived in/accessibility of existing NHS installations in or near the District.
> Aspects of health services most important to the service user.
> Over what aspects of health services do the target populations wish to have a choice?
> Alternative means of accessing NHS services.
> Importance attached to location of a health service compared with its other aspects characteristics.
> What locations for health services do the target populations prefer? Why?

sense of promoting NHS services to potential users is a corollary for sellers with volume-based contracts (including GP contracts) but also a different activity, explained in the next section. Selling in the sense considered now is akin to industrial not consumer selling and in the NHS internal markets will occur in two main forms.

Selling large-scale health services within the internal market

This is the concern of SGTs, GPs selling secondary care, and DMUs insofar as service contracting is administered in ways which make them imitate the SGTs. SGTs will have to sell their services both to buyers and to GPs with practice budgets. For these sellers three main practical questions are who should do the selling, what sales promotion media they should use, and how the quality of an NHS service can be presented as a selling point.

In answer to the question of who should do the selling US experience suggests that for major contracts the CEO or UGM is the most suitable salesperson.[7] (In the NHS 'major' contracts will be those with DHAs or RHAs, rather than contracts with GPs holding practice budgets.) The CEO will however require the following support; in effect the SGT's sales team.

- Clinical advisers (e.g. DPHs, Medical Directors, epidemiologists) and quality assurance managers to present and negotiate details of the quality specification.
- Financial staff to present the pricing and payment terms possible incentives or penalties.
- Marketers to present any market research on which the proposed service specification is based and to make more detailed presentations using the media noted below.
- Advisers on any legal or drafting technicalities of proposed contracts.
- It may also be prudent to introduce whoever would be the day-to-day point of liaison for tracking, problem-solving and other servicing purposes should the contract be awarded. The CEO, or the salesperson representing the CEO, can supplement this with information on the contract servicing and evaluation.

The question of what sales promotion media to use comes next. Given the complexity and the technical nature of the negotiations, together with the need for flexibility and negotiation over details, personal selling, conferences and seminars are likelier to be more effective methods of presenting a proposed service than conventional advertising. This can be done through one-to-one meetings, formal presentations or site visits. Personal contact can be used to develop these and generate a feeling of personal obligation to the seller as adverts cannot[8] and is likely to be the major channel for selling to DHAs.

However, service contracts will presumably have to be let under HA standing orders and other NHS financial regulations. This may limit the scope for personal selling as a means for gaining preferential treatment in securing service contracts. Against this, it is theoretically possible to interpret tendering procedures in ways that limit competition if for some reason the buyer wishes to enter a bilateral relationship with one favoured seller. An obvious way is to make the favoured seller's unique selling points the criterion for eligibility to tender for the contract. This will limit the number of eligible providers to one. For selling to GPs with practice budgets (a large number of small purchasers) formal presentations (workshops, seminars or 'conferences'), perhaps combined with material incentives, are probably the most effective medium.

There are three main steps in using service quality as a selling point:

- Discover what quality issues the HAs and GPs wish to contract for. These issues are of two kinds. For HAs there is the mix of services, and the quality specification for each which the buyer will stipulate for its particular District. What the buyer's intentions are in this matter can only be answered empirically by market research, using the methods outlined in Chapter 4 to address the questions mentioned at step 5B and in Table 4.1. However there are secondly a number of seller characteristics which all buyers interested in maintaining service quality would rationally insist upon. As these are defined from the buyer's viewpoint they are considered at step 14, p. 121.
- Ensure that the seller can credibly claim to be able to provide services of this quality. This requires the seller either to demonstrate this capacity from existing services, or be able to demonstrate that it has the managerial capacity to implement the remaining steps of the marketing cycle (especially steps 18, 21 to 26), and the physical resources to do so. Accreditation is one way of showing the latter.
- Present these claims to the buyers. This step resembles conventional commercial selling and can be outlined by reinterpreting for the NHS internal market a standard marketing model of selling.

Various texts expand upon these models and the practical skills of salesmanship[9]. In these models the main stages in selling are:

- Prospecting for potential buyers. This involves identifying organizations likely to wish to buy services of the kind the seller sells, and within these organizations identifying the individuals or groups who take the buying decision. It remains unclear exactly how DHAs will be structured for these purposes but it is reasonable to assume that major buying decisions will be taken by the GMs or even the HA itself on GM recommendation.
- Contacting the buyers. In selling to commercial organizations it is advantageous to have some pretext for approaching potential buyers which sets one apart from the numerous salesmen that many commercial managers are solicited by (e.g. a common extra-mural interest). In the NHS in the early 1990s most existing NHS managers will be able to draw upon the working links built up before the internal market and their professional organizations in contacting influential individuals.

Vignette 5.1   The Manchester clinic: a market niche

In the middle 1980s Manchester Royal Infirmary (MRI) had many medical staff who undertook private practice at nearby commercial hospitals. The MRI also had a Private Patients Home which was in need of refurbishment and financial review and lay nearer the city centre and main transport routes than the commercial hospitals. Central Manchester HA saw scope to capitalize on this combination of circumstances. The Private Patients Home was refurbished and established as the 34-bed Manchester Clinic, a managerially independent enterprise in competition with other commercial health services. Initially the Manchester Clinic had its own medical directorship but management of the clinic was seen contracted to UME, and later became a joint Health Authority–UME activity.

Its unique selling points to patients were its connections with a teaching hospital for Europe's largest medical school and the availability of clinical support services unmatched by any commercial hospital (suggesting high clinical standards). Its hotel services were positioned at a level higher than normal NHS provision in the MRI but not as expensive as those in independent for-profit hospitals. For medical staff the venture's unique selling point was opportunity for private practice without the inconvenience of working between two or more sites and (again) full back-up services. The new service opened in 1986 and has established itself as one of the city's main ventures for private practice. It is targeted to earn a seven-figure profit in the 1989–1990 financial year.

- Introducing the service which the seller wishes to sell, seeking to relate its selling points as far as possible to the buyer's interests rather than the seller's. In the internal market, it will be necessary for sellers to be able to claim that the service they offer has some unique selling point to distinguish it from NHS and other competitors. For many DGHs their location, the fact that they have been designed as a local monopoly provider and the convenience of retaining existing referral patterns, infrastructure and management links will be important USPs. However there are other ways that NHS providers can differentiate themselves from both NHS and commercial competitors, as Vignette 5.1 illustrates.
- Deal with buyer objections or resistances. Flexibility and sensitivity to the buyer's demands is required as is the ability to avoid either pressuring the buyer too obviously or underselling the service.
- 'Close' the sale, having negotiated any variations on the quality specification to meet the buyer's demands.

Selling income-generating services also requires some selling point to differentiate the NHS income-generator from the many income-generators (primarily salesmen) from other intending suppliers by whom the potential NHS customer will also be lobbied. Service differentiation is harder for competitors to match, especially differentiation based on staff competences, image and the social dimension of care.[10] Buildings, equipment, promotional materials or other 'hardware' are copied easily.

Price and cost will be a major selling consideration but here only the marketing effects of pricing are relevant. The price of a service may be interpreted as an indicator of its quality. Too low a price may raise doubts as to how such a quality of service can be provided. (To use low or under-pricing as a selling point is therefore risky in marketing as well as in financial terms.) Within the restrictions of commercial confidentiality an overview of the seller's costings can be used to help relieve such anxieties. Prices can also be set high to deter the sale of services which an SGT may feel obliged to offer for public relations reasons but are unprofitable or are unattractive for other reasons.

'Income generation' in the sense of sales of 'extras' and excess capacity by DMUs, for instance the optional extras for hospital patients recommended in *Working For Patients*, is the second main arena for selling. The internal market will make this a secondary, but still an important, commercial activity for NHS organizations. Methods of market research for income generation are still under-researched.[11] However ideas for generating income can be found in:

- The managerial literature (e.g. *Health Services Journal*, *Health Services Management*) occasionally report commercially successful ventures.
- Specialist consultants. Vignette 5.2 gives one consultant's list of offerings.
- Directories sold by Health Authorities such as Central Manchester (as an income-generating venture!).
- Exhibitions such as IGEX.

For generating secondary income there are four main 'customer' segments:

- Commercial and industrial 'customers', including other NHS organizations. These are likely to be interested primarily in commercial benefits (in kind or cash) and secondarily in public relations benefits. For instance a firm may wish to offer certain groups of its employees health screening as a fringe benefit but not at the prices charged by commercial health screening providers. Firms outside the NHS may see a public relations bonus in being associated with such a popular institution. The selling methods here are much the same as for service contracts (see p. 116).

Vignette 5.2 Income generation in Health Authorities; 52 ways

Health Authorities are discovering increasingly diverse ways to supplement their income from the Department of Health and a number of consultancies now offer assistance. One consultancy alone offers advice on the following methods of income generation:

Advertising contained in appointment cards

Advertising on hospital walls
Advertising in hospital publications
Bank facilities
Book clubs
Car boot sales
Car parking facilities
Charitable payroll giving
Chemists (franchises on hospital sites)
Coffee shop catering
Convenience foods
Contracting
Development of shopping facilities
Discounts on travel for staff and Health Authority members
Drug stores
Dry cleaning
Training agency grants
EEC grants
Estate agency
Facilities for solicitors
Grants for charities, private limited companies and trusts
Guzzler Puzzlers – Children's and adult puzzles
Health food shops
Health promotion
Health screening
Healthy snacks
Hire of phones for patients
Hire of TVs for patients
Holiday travel discounts
Income from wills
Insurance companies
Joint ventures with the private sector
Sale of laundry services to the community and private sector
Management buyouts
Newsagents
Opticians
Photographic processing
Poster advertising
Promotion of lotteries
Sale of aids for the disabled
Sale of catering services
Sale of clinical services to private sector and nursing homes
Sale of commemorative plaques in maternity units
Sale of land
Silver recovery
Shops in maternity units
Sub post office
Telephone services
Travel agents
Travel clinics
Weekend markets in hospital car parks.

Source: Colin M. Barnett Associates PLC.

- Public funding bodies outside the Department of Health, for instance the EEC and the various parts of the DTI and Department of Employment who fund training, retraining and work creation schemes. Discovering the formal, published criteria for eligibility for funding through these bodies is comparatively straightforward. What is harder, but critical to success of applications, is to know the unpublished criteria and policy agendas by which grants are allocated. Various consultancies can advise but many demand as much as 10% of the cash obtained.
- Charitable donors. NHS organizations have continued to accept charitable donations ever since 1947 but legal changes in 1980 made scope for them to seek donations more actively. On US experience, firms tend to avoid donating to controversial causes (but most NHS activity is uncontroversial) and prefer to donate locally.[12] Experience suggests that the most effective images for public fundraising for individuals represent health care as acute curative care, often with high technology, provided for the more attractive client groups such as babies or (respectable) elderly people. By contrast, promoting community care requires emphasis on non-curative social care for socially marginal groups, some of whom (e.g. the mentally disordered) are often regarded as deviant or dangerous. This problem will become more acute if NHS organizations take advantage of the IBA's recent decision to increase the scope for charitable advertising on television. US experience also suggests that in seeking donations from rich individuals the most profitable route is to concentrate on the highly-educated, middle-aged stratum.[13] This may be harder to achieve in Britain, where public displays of wealth and generosity are apparently not considered as acceptable as they are in the USA. Identifying rich donors (besides those who have already donated) is made difficult by the fact that income is a personal detail respondents are most reluctant to disclose to market researchers. What motivates wealthy donors may be public recognition, desire to serve the public interest or to be publicly associated with one's social betters.[14]
- Direct sales to the public. Here conventional advertising and selling methods have the greatest applicability. In health care the public may perceive price as an indicator of quality and think (wrongly) that health services they pay for are of higher quality than free services.[15]

Many health authorities still have a once-off competitive advantage in being able to decide when, and with what product, they enter new markets. They have the disadvantage of inexperience and a limited proven record of providing services under commercial conditions. Government policy sometimes compounds these disadvantages. For example, central policy has in recent years been for the NHS to sell surplus land and buildings when it would be more in NHS interests to rent or lease if possible; that way the NHS would still gain income from the land or buildings but also retain ownership of a rapidly appreciating asset. In any event the decision arises of whether to try to compete on a price or a non-price basis, i.e. to develop income-generating activities whose unique selling point is high value for money or a real characteristic of the product (e.g. the expertise of the staff providing it, or the opportunity to support the NHS).

Step 14. Buyers select providers

In practice NHS buyers' selection of providers will depend on a range of largely non-marketing objectives outlined in the business plan, such as cost, the financial soundness of SGTs and compliance with central health policy. In practice the providers of non-core services are more likely to be sellers than the providers of core services, but even the providers of non-core services could in principle be extra-territorial DMUs. There are already examples of this arrangement in the NHS. But there are further marketing questions for NHS buyers to ask of sellers seeking service contracts:

- Has the provider presented trackable and achievable quality specifications for both the clinical and the non-clinical dimensions of the service? (Compare Table 3.5.)
- How do these specifications compare with equivalent specifications offered by other providers? This is the critical question, especially in regard to the clinical dimensions of care.
- Is the provider developing and using outcome indicators?
- Has the provider developed a marketing, market research and tracking infrastructure, and in which specialties? (The Deparament of Health appear to attach special weight to whether clinical audit is used for tracking.) Do the seller's prices appear to allow for the cost of this infrastructure and of tracking?
- How regularly does the provider conduct market research and evaluations? What use is made of the results?
- How much support does the provider give to service innovations, research and development, and staff education training; i.e. how is its range of services likely to develop?
- Is the provider willing to seek accreditation when available?
- What does the buyer's own market research reveal about the reputation the provider has with experienced users, disinterested expert advisers, GPs and care managers and the mass media?
- If the provider is an SGT, what balance does it strike between pursuing commercial and health objectives?
- How well developed are the provider's health promotion, intersectoral and preventive activities (where applicable)?
- Will the provider allow the buyer unforewarned access to premises, patients and records?
- What record of achieving quality and marketing objectives do the provider's past tracking data show?
- What procedures and practice has the provider for remedying problems and complaints?

On the buyer's side, the pursuit of innovation requires a broad, imaginative view of forms of service to consider buying and of possible providers. It would be quite legitimate for a DHA or GP with a practice budget to approach, say, housing organizations to provide long-term care for elderly chronically-ill people or pressure groups or professional lobbyists to pursue health promotion, intersectoral or health policy objectives.[16] In a seller's market it may also become necessary for the buyer to promote itself as an organization worthwhile to win contracts from. Lastly some services may prove more profitable, or attractive to sellers for other reasons, than others (for instance cold surgery is likely to yield a more predictable profit than major accident cover can). If this creates difficulty finding sellers of some services, the buyer may wish to consider bundling these services with more commercially attractive services, making it a condition for awarding a contract for the latter that the seller also provide the former. In this case special attention would have to be paid to tracking the less 'attractive' service.

Step 15. Negotiating the contract

For buyers the critical marketing task is to negotiate the contract in such a way that ensures the seller can and must meet the buyer's service quality specification. For sellers the corresponding task is to ensure that their commercial objectives are satisfied. In negotiating the contract, marketing considerations will in practice have to be weighed against non-marketing considerations (the legalities, cost, etc.) although the Department of Health evidently intends that quality considerations should be given greater weight than cost in service contracting. They also appear to intend the buyers to open the bidding and to keep the initiative in negotiating quality specifications. This will be practicable for the buyers if the type of service quality specification described in Chapter 3 is used as the basis for service contract negotiations and (presumably modified in the negotiations) for the service contract itself.

A main concern for buyers will be to ensure that the contract identifies the substantive tracking variables and the levels which would trigger further investigation or other action (see Chapter 3, step 10, p. 69 and Chapter 6, step 23, p. 161). For buyers to be able to track the services they buy, the contract must allow buyer access to the seller's medical records and administrative records relevant to tracking variables (e.g. waiting intervals from GP referral to first hospital attendance). The seller would presumably wish for the medical records normally to be anonymized for this purpose and to allow access only to administrative information that was not commercially confidential for other reasons. Similarly the buyer would be prudent to seek rights of access to the seller's premises (or at least, those areas where patients and public have free access) and to the patients themselves. Experience with the Health and Safety Executive and other inspectorates suggest that these rights of access would most effectively serve the buyer's tracking purposes if the contract stated that they could be exercised without prior warning to the

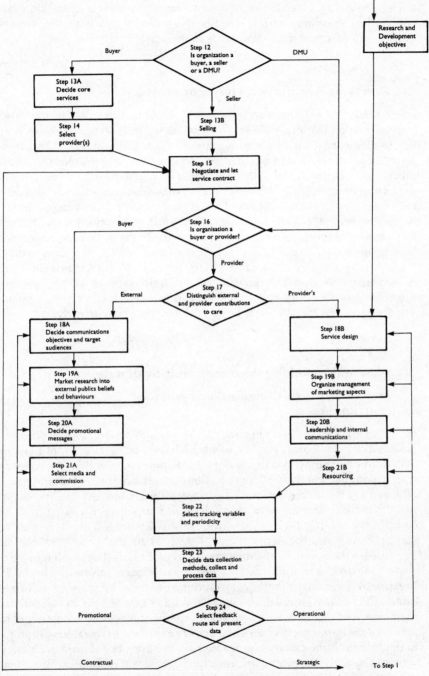

Figure 5.1 The NHS marketing process: marketing mix and implementation phases

seller. The contract would also have to define the ownership of tracking data collected in this way, stating whether the buyer would have the right to publish any of it, and if so under what conditions.

Step 16. Is organization a buyer or provider?

Implementation of a marketing strategy proceeds differently in the NHS internal market for buyers and providers. As the next section explains (step 17) implementing an NHS marketing strategy requires two concurrent activities of service design and delivery (on one hand) and promotion (on the other). The essence of the NHS internal market is that the buyers contract out the service design and delivery to providers organizationally distinct from the buyer, not undertake these themselves. A concomitant of providing a service is that the providers have to target 'operational' promotions towards their service users (besides salesmanship towards the buyers). But the buyers too have promotional objectives and activities of their own (e.g. to demonstrate publicly how they have discharged their duties, explain their priorities and decisions, to respond to criticism, etc.). The buyers' marketing activity therefore proceeds only down the left hand branch out of step 16 in Figure 5.1; the providers' marketing follows both branches concurrently.

Promotions: deciding the communication strategy

Step 17. Distinguish external and provider contributions to care

Health care is inherently a joint activity by a health service with its patients, informal carers and other publics, of whom buyers are the most important for SGTs. Implementing health services marketing correspondingly has two major, complementary components. For each service the contribution each of these agents makes to care can be identified from the quality chain, identified from market research as described in Chapter 3 (step 7). The contribution of the NHS organization is made through the activities of service design and the deployment of staff, estate and other resources as described in the internal implementation part of the flow diagram (Figure 5.1, steps 18B, 19B, 20B and 21B), as the next chapter explains. The NHS organization can manage the contribution made by the patients, informal carers, the healthy population, buyers and other external publics (insofar as their contribution can be managed at all) through its promotional strategy, to influence the opinions, decisions and behaviours of the external contributors. In practice both the external (promotional) and the internal implementation activities have to take place concurrently. Text, however, cannot but present them in sequence and Figure 5.1 gives a more accurate picture than the textual sequence can of how the external promotional activity described in this

Table 5.2 NHS and external users' contributions to health care; a worked example from the part of the quality chain for an outpatients department illustrated in Figure 3.3

GP
    Decision to refer to secondary care
    Choice of secondary care provider to refer to
    Decision on what services to seek from secondary provider (e.g. whether for tests only, tests and opinion, out-patient treatment, admission, etc.)

Patient
    Agreement with GP's recommendation to refer
    Acceptance or modification of GP's choice of secondary provider to refer to
    Acceptance of OPD appointment offer and active reply
    Toleration of waiting time
    Arranges time off work, babysitting, care for other dependants etc. for visit to OPD
    Travels to hospital, finds OPD, presents him/herself to reception
    Compliance with receptionist's instructions
    Consents to tests and complies with test procedure
    Tolerates waits in OPD
    Consents to doctor's examination and complies with its procedures
    Accepts or modifies proposed treatment plan, etc.

Informal carer
    Helps with the journey to hospital
    Helps explain the procedure to the patient, reassures him/her
    Tolerates wait for the patient's tests, consultation, etc.

Voluntary hospital workers
    Provide transport to hospital
    Provide refreshments and guidance in OPD waiting area

chapter has to be co-ordinated with the internal implementation described in Chapter 6.

Table 5.2 identifies the audiences and contributions to care embodied in the part quality chain illustrated in Figure 3.3.

Step 18A. Decide Promotion objectives and target audiences

'Promotions' are all activities by which an organization influences the beliefs and behaviour of its various 'customers'. In the NHS, 'customer' has to be interpreted widely to refer to patients, carers and the other groups listed below. For GPs, sellers and DMUs who accept cost and volume and case-cost based service contracts, NHS marketing differs from standard commercial marketing in that their cash income depends on attracting patients not only upon influencing the buyers. For these organizations promotional activity is always on two fronts, towards users and towards buyers. In the NHS internal market there are three kinds of promotional objective. One is predominantly the concern of providers and can be called 'operational' promotion. 'Strategic' and 'user-led' promotion objectives are common to all NHS organizations.

The operational promotion objectives of an NHS provider are to get the external contributors to health care (see Table 5.2) to make the contribution required in the way that most effectively meets the NHS organization's objectives. The relevant events in the quality chain for these promotional purposes are those corresponding to what Chapter 3 called the 'necessarily user-led' service characteristics. Here promotional activity complements the quality specification and service design (see step 18B). The quality specification states, and service design meets, the requirements which the users set as a condition for taking up the service or for compliance; external promotions let users know this has been done. The common question: 'How to produce promotional materials such as patient handbooks or practice leaflets?' can be answered by showing how producing operational promotions parallels, and how it differs from, producing a quality specification and service design. Because of the close connection with line management, the obvious person to take charge of producing operational promotions is the department head or clinical director of the service concerned. For buyer organizations, strategic objectives will preponderate but even they may have some operational promotional objectives, for instance to influence external contributors to the quality chain to influence patterns of referral and self-referral (e.g. to reduce cross-boundary flow or encourage uptake of preventive services provided by GPs or other providers contracted directly to the DHA).

Strategic promotion objectives comprise intersectoral planning objectives (e.g. to persuade local authorities to provide more housing for single people), health policy objectives (e.g. to persuade government to tax alcohol more heavily) and image-building beyond that required for immediate operational purposes. These communications are most suitably managed by the DGM or UGM (or the equivalent) or, in the case of health promotion and intersectoral promotions, by a specialist department.

'User-led' communication objectives are simply the provision of whatever information NHS users want, irrespective of whether this coincides with the operational or strategic communications objectives. In the terminology of Chapter 3, these objectives are 'rationally user-led' because the service users can be presumed to know best what information they happen to want.

Internal promotions aimed at provider organizations' staff, are considered in Chapter 6 as part of the internal implementation process. However, most of the practical considerations which apply to external promotions also apply to internal promotions. The main promotional activity towards buyers is salesmanship, which has already been considered (step 13B – see Fig 5.1 and p. 113) but towards which the practical considerations below also apply.

Objectives for operational and the strategic promotions alike can be formulated in behavioural or in attitudinal terms. User-led requirements for information are formulated purely in attitudinal terms. Behavioural objectives state what 'customer' behaviours a communications strategy is to promote. These will include the behaviours necessary for achieving the NHS organization's objectives (see Chapter 3, step 1, p. 46). Examples:

- To achieve 98% takeup of cervical cancer screening services by women aged 30–45 resident in the DHA by the end of 1992.
- To attract at least 100 000 GP referrals for cold surgery during the current service contract period.
- To expand the practice list to 12 000 patients by 31 December 1990.

Attitudinal objectives are to influence target audiences' knowledge of health care (including self-care), the image they have of the NHS organization, and their opinions on health policy matters. It is often supposed that a target audience's knowledge directly influences its behaviour. However this assumption is certainly simplistic and may even reverse the actual relationship. (It can be argued that individuals change their opinions as a consequence of changed behaviour or circumstances, to rationalize the former and to 'explain' the latter.[17]) Beliefs are however easier to change by promotional means than behaviours are, as the effect of public health campaigns on AIDS illustrates.[18] User requirements for knowledge were described as a 'rationally user-led' service characteristic in Chapter 3 (step 8, p. 66) and this suggests that a second type of attitudinal objective would be to use promotions to meet this need. Examples of attitudinal objectives might include:

- To rectify the damage done to the image of the NHS and DHAs by the *Working for Patients* proposals.[19]
- To reduce the stigmatizing effects of prejudice against the mentally handicapped.
- To raise to 51% or more the proportion of responding DHA residents who support water fluoridation.
- To inform patients of the range of services available at X hospital or general practice.
- To give a general explanation of what cataracts are, how they are treated, and how patients and their families can assist the hospital.

External target audiences for the strategic promotions can be identified from the business plan and from the quality chain for intersectoral activity, health promotion and health education activities. Target audiences for operational promotions can be derived directly from the quality chain. In most NHS cases the main target audiences will include:

- Those directly involved in care; patients, informal carers, co-providers (other agencies including other NHS groups e.g. GPs, LASS, etc.), blood and organ donors. These can be identified from the quality chain, from the business plan, contract and service specification.
- Sources of referrals. For general practice, A&E services, some forms of social care and other points of first resort this source will be the service user

Table 5.3 Operational promotional objectives associated with the part quality chain outlined in Figure 3.3

---

1 To attract GP referrals for the full range of hospital services (opinion, diagnosis, in-patient and out-patient treatment, rehabilitation) by assuring GPs of the speed and quality of the clinical work offered.

2 To attract patients to refer themselves to the hospital (via A&E and outreach clinics) or to ask their GPs to refer them to this hospital and OPD, by assuring patients of the quality of care at this hospital, and by informing patients of whatever attributes the OPD service are likely to attract them.

3 To provide the information about the OPD and about clinical care that is necessary to meet the patients' and GPs' own information needs, and in forms which are intelligible to patients and GPs.

4 To provide the information necessary to enable patients to reach the OPD, at the places and times they require in forms which are intelligible to them.

5 To provide the information necessary to enable patients and informal carers to make full use of the hospital's services once they are referred or admitted.

6 To recruit voluntary workers and informal carers.

7 To recruit donors of organs, blood, etc.·

---

or relatives. For secondary services it is the GP or the care manager, for tertiary services other hospital doctors.

● Health promotional audiences, including intersectoral audiences, health-related industries. These can be identified from *Health For All 2000* and its supporting documents, health profiles and health policy documents besides the quality chains for preventive, health promotion and health education services.

● Health policy audiences; the political establishments, the general public and pressure groups such as MIND. NHS organizations are likeliest to encounter political opposition and controversy in addressing the last two targets. For moral reasons, for example, Mrs Thatcher has reputedly encouraged a 'pussy-footing' rather than a direct approach to sex education about AIDS.[20]

Table 5.3 gives worked example analysing the part quality chain shown in Figure 3.3 to differentiate these objectives.

Step 19B. Market research into user and public beliefs, behaviours

To discover the messages and media likely to achieve the promotional objectives requires market research (see Table 4.1). Chapter 4 outlines possible methods of market research, here used to reconstruct empirically the beliefs and motives that influence whether or how the target audiences contribute to the provision of care. This is the NHS analogue to the examination of buying decisions and buying behaviours of individual consumers in conventional marketing theory. Since the NHS service user is not a buyer research in health services management, the psychology of health and illness and in medical sociology may shed more light on NHS user's beliefs and behaviour than most secondary research in marketing can. These sources can be accessed via libraries and databases as described in Chapters 3 and 4. The market research is also used to investigate how target audiences' beliefs on health matters are formed. Here the focus is to discover what users think the NHS organization is actually like rather than (as in specifying quality) what they think it ought to be like. The 'beliefs' to research include the image that a particular care group have of health care or the NHS, 'image' being taken to mean 'the totality of beliefs about, and attitudes towards' the service or patient group in question.

To set objectives for operational promotions, the market research will have to investigate the user decisions that occur in the quality chain and what attitudinal factors influence them. For instance:

- Why do people seek health care (e.g. for the relief of symptoms, for relief of anxiety, to talk to a GP about emotional problems, to legitimate withdrawal from work or other social activity?)? Why do clients seek social care?
- What degree of knowledge or recall of existence of a particular service do its potential users (or their GPs) have?
- What reputation does the practice or hospital have? What do potential users think the best and the worst aspects of the general practice or the hospital?
- Where would the target population first think to turn for health care of a given kind?
- Which members of the household influence the patient's choice of a source of health or social care?
- For non-urgent care, how do users co-ordinate their uptake of health services with other daily activities? (For example, is a visit to the GP fitted in with the next shopping trip or lunchtime at work? Do users assume that going to the doctor always requires a special trip out?)
- How do users select their health service providers? What quality issues (i.e. what service characteristics) attract referrals or self-referrals?
- What deters potential users from taking up a particular service? (e.g. why are so many people afraid of dentistry?)
- How do they differentiate it or 'position' it against the alternatives? How do the target audiences respond to competitors' promotions?
- What other general practices or hospitals do they see as alternatives?
- Why do people donate blood or organs voluntarily?

To assist in setting the strategic promotional objectives the market research will have to investigate such questions as:

- What do the target audiences know about what diseases are preventable?
- Do they know what health behaviours and self-care can reduce their risk?

- What image do people have of the NHS, how it should be run, the level of funding it requires, etc?
- Are these images favourable or hostile?
- How much confidence do the target audiences have in the efficacy of NHS care?
- What expectations do public have of NHS services and medical technologies, and of the role of the NHS?
- What can be done to encourage the dissemination and uptake of new types of service? A standard marketing model analyses the process of dissemination and uptake of new services into four phases, in each of which a distinct segment of the user population are the main converts. Figure 5.2 illustrates this.[21] Market research can then be used to identify 'selling' points to each of these segments, and their likely resistances so that the content of the promotional methods can be targeted accordingly.

To find the user-led objectives the market researcher has simply to ask users (perhaps with prompting) what information about NHS services or health care they want.

For selecting the media for communicating with the target audiences it is also necessary to find out where the public and patients turn for information about health matters, which media influence their opinions in health matters, which media have the highest credibility on health matters and how the answers to these questions differ for different segments of the target audiences. This is another market research task. Secondary research data suggests that almost any NHS promotional strategy will require a segmentation of its target audiences. It has already been shown, for instance, that blue-collar workers place less confidence in medical care than white-collar workers do

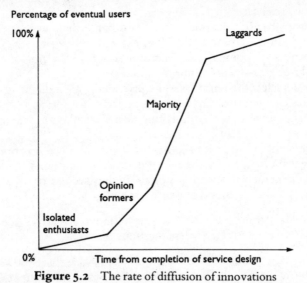

Figure 5.2 The rate of diffusion of innovations

Source: Adapted from Ashton and Seymour, *The New Public Health* (1988), Open University Press

and respond differently to illness.[22] In that case, materials encouraging workers to take up screening services may have to use different emphases and presentational media to the two groups.

Communications: messages and media

Step 21A. Decide promotional messages

The results of the market research can be used in two ways to decide what messages the NHS organization should prioritize. User-led information requirements can be read off directly from the market research findings. But users' attitudes and behaviours do not have to be taken uncritically. The point of NHS promotions is to influence and alter these beliefs e.g. to disabuse unrealistic expectations that medical technology or the NHS cannot satisfy, educate and explain the NHS role to public, explain priorities and decisions. Operational and strategic promotion objectives are derived from comparing the target audiences' actual knowledge and behaviours with what are necessary to meet the NHS organization's requirements. Promotional activity is then targeted on reducing any gaps. A standard method for operational purposes is to suggest that services can indeed offer benefits which the users seek (e.g. by offering GPs prompt results from pathology tests or from requests for opinion) or to allay any fears (e.g. by reminding elderly patients that they will probably be exempt from any charges). These will probably become standard advertising tactics of SGTs. For operational purposes the substance of the message is derived from market research evidence about what features of an NHS service encourage or deter uptake. For strategic purposes the message is chosen to correct the most important gaps in knowledge of self-care or the NHS indicated by market research or to contest any negative images of the NHS, promote healthier behaviours or NHS views on health policy. This is how an NHS organization can get its consumers to make 'informed choices' about what services can and should be offered.

What substantive messages are required thus depends above all on the contingent findings of market research. Nevertheless a few generalizations are possible. A standard marketing formula recommends that a successful promotional medium gains attention, arouses interest, creates a desire for the product, service or policy objective, and stimulates action to get it. Enlarging Clarke and Kotler's suggestions,[23] it appears that NHS messages are likeliest to overcome any audience resistance when they:

- Offer something desirable, in terms of the audience's own preferences (whether an advantageous service or a desirable health policy objective). It has long been known that messages which try to frighten people into seeking health care are comparatively ineffective.[24] (Compare: 'Don't die of ignorance'.)
- Present a message or offer a service which is distinctive to the sender (e.g. when a general practice offers a weekend service which no other local

practice can). Also the presentation must be distinctive to grasp attention in the face of many competitors.

- Be credible, and if possible presented by a credible, well-known figure.
- Have a form of presentation consistent with the stated message. For instance a mission statement or video announcing a DHA's concern with quality is less likely to look convincing if it looks amateurish and scrappy.
- Present a defensible message; one that is true (not half-truth), non-vacuous and non-trivial. A negative example is a recent TV advert claiming that a major private health company is non profit-making; this is true of its insurance activities but not of its hospital services. One aspect of this, in the areas of health policy and intersectoral planning, is to anticipate and disable possible counter-promotions from other organizations. In the case of caring services, a defensible message is one that only promises what the NHS organization can in fact provide.

The ethics of the proposed message should also be considered. The debates noted in Chapter 3 make it worth asking how far NHS promotions can legitimately exploit emotional or non-rational messages (e.g. 'Safe sex is fun'). Health promoters sometimes come under pressure to soften messages about health behaviours, reducing a possibly life-saving impact on the target audience, to placate public opinion or the prejudices of great personages. (Mrs Thatcher has reportedly delayed and diluted HEA advertising on AIDS to the point of ineffectiveness.)[25] A health promotion message used to reduce the damage of unhealthy behaviours (e.g. to encourage drug users to accept clean exchange needles) may be taken as condoning illegal or immoral behaviour; but this may be a price worth paying if it saves lives.

Vignette 5.3   A preferred caseload

Mr B is a general dental practitioner in a coastal city. Partly out of personal taste and partly because of the structure of NHS payments for GP dentistry in 1989, Mr B preferred a caseload with a high proportion of high-income families with young children and single adults, preferably in white-collar occupations. His other preferred segment of patients are career women aged 30–50 who practice good dental self-care. (The fact that he has these preferences suggests that Mr B has already done a rudimentary form of business planning and market research on his possible areas of activity.) From his local knowledge Mr B already knew where his preferred clientele tended to live, the shops and garages they tended to use and what newsagents and local papers served these areas. He has used petrol stations and the Post Office service for mass delivery to householders to make his practice known in areas likely to be inhabited by the sorts of patient he wishes to recruit. Like most other patients Mr B's preferred clientele place at least as much value on the social acceptability of the dentist's finished work-manship and on the practitioner's interactive manner and skills as upon his technical standard of dental work.

Source: 'Market Forces – Packaging the Professions', BBC Radio 4.

Messages communicated by NHS organizations can be straightforwardly positive promotion of services, health behaviours or health policy. This is the closest analogue to commercial promotions and advertising. Vignette 5.3 is an NHS example.

However they can also use the approaches of social marketing, demarketing and anti-marketing. 'Social marketing' consists, for NHS purposes, in using marketing and promotional techniques to advance a social or political objective, for example to 'explain the reasons' for *Working for Patients*. Vignette 5.4 shows some factors behind the BMA's recent success at social marketing on this issue. Similar methods, citing tracking and health planning data, can be used by a DHA to promulgate messages about what it has achieved and how it has discharged its public duties.

Social marketing requires a heavy reliance on news media, 'events' (e.g. the ambulancemen's record-breaking petition) and outreach to other organizations, for instance to recruit the support of pressure groups, professional bodies and celebrities. It is critical to try to set the terms of the debate, and hence to try to keep the initiative in social marketing activity and messages. It is necessary to sustain the activity over a long period and periodically publish evidence of support.

Demarketing uses the same techniques but to deter service uptake. This is occasionally legitimate, for instance when encouraging people with minor injuries to use GPs rather than hospital accident and emergency services, or discouraging mobile patients from using over-stretched ambulance services, or *ad hoc* during industrial action or rebuilding schemes. However the dangers of delaying health care (or deterring it altogether) make demarketing a riskier strategy in the NHS than elsewhere. If demarketing is to be used, an obvious precaution is to place the onus on the manager or clinician recommending it to establish that no harm will thereby be done to patients.

Demarketing is only ever a partial reversal of positive promotion; even staff who must turn patients away still have to be trained to do this civilly and with a clear explanation of the reason. Clarke and Kotler's recommendation that messages offer something desirable to the audience (see above) suggests that the most effective way to demarket one service would be to promote the alternative most likely to appeal to its users (e.g. to reduce pressure on ambulances by promoting the hospital's minibus and voluntary car services or demarket the cottage hospital by promoting the DGH). Besides communication media, pricing can be used to demarket services (e.g. charging for the replacement of negligently lost or damaged aids or appliances). In normally free services almost any pricing is likely to have some deterrent effects.[26] The effects of demarketing must be restricted as far as possible only to deterring unsuitable patients, not those for whom the service is intended (e.g. serious accident victims). This makes targeting the demarketing activities upon clearly-defined segments and tracking the results particularly important.

Anti-marketing consists of using communications techniques to subvert the marketing of organizations trying to sell sickness-causing products such

---

Vignette 5.4   An SOS for the NHS

Following the damage to its reputation in the disputes over NHS pay beds and doctors contracts in the 1970s, the BMA has modernized its approach to public relations, concentrating on health policy issues and presenting itself as a patients' advocate rather than as a professional interest group. This strategy has been applied through the BMA's media division. For journalists this offers a contact service, providing names of experts on medical and health policy matters so that journalists find it easy and quick to use the BMA media division as a source for copy. The service relies on a bibliographical database and medical contact list. The same approach was next applied to MPs, on whose views and interests the BMA also runs a computerized database (as much a resource for its members to use in lobbying as an aid to the press).

In 1989 a campaign against *Working for Patients* drew upon the goodwill that had accumulated. Five main media for publicity and for placing pressure on MPs were used. To sustain attention and effect, each of these were used in sequence. Doctors were first urged to write to their MPs (many did). An advertising campaign (mainly posters and leaflets for patients) followed, with production and distribution of posters sub-contracted to an advertising agency. The main poster slogan was 'What do you call a man who ignores medical advice? – Kenneth Clarke', that on the leaflets 'An SOS for the NHS'. In each constituency the leaflet named the local MP. Two opinion polls were next commissioned, and tending to support the BMA's case, were publicised as media events timed to coincide with the periodic reappearance of the White Paper on parliamentary agendas. As media events, public meetings were held region by region, targeting both urban and rural areas. All this followed the Department of Health's own promotion of *Working for Patients*, putting the Government in the position of being able at most to complain about the content of the BMA's messages but hardly about BMA methods.

Sources: Timmins, N. 'Massive Dose of Persuasion', *Independent* 20 July 1989. British Medical Association *An SOS for the NHS* (Leaflet). Young, H. 'Learning to Play Dirty in the Health Wars' *Guardian* 31 August 1989.

---

as tobacco and high-cholesterol foods. Shielding the NHS organization from possible legal consequences can either be achieved by sheer ingenuity, as Vignette 5.5 illustrates, or by discretely assisting independent pressure groups such as the Billboard-Utilizing Graffiti Artists Against Unhealthy Promotions, (BUGAAUHP; the acronym more or less describes what they do to tobacco adverts, for instance by over-spraying them with such slogans as 'Their gold, your lungs').[27] For obvious reasons 'anti-marketing' is considered disreputable by most trade organizations in advertising and marketing but is altogether too useful for health promotion, intersectoral planning and health policy campaigns for health managers to ignore.

Social marketing, and anti-marketing even more, are likely to provoke counter-advertising or other counter-promotions. An important contributor to the defensibility of a social marketing or anti-marketing message is its ability to pre-empt or neutralize the more obvious replies. NHS health

Vignette 5.5   Anti-marketing tobacco: project smoke-free

Young consumers are critical of the future of the tobacco industry; their early addiction to tobacco generates its long-term income. Although tobacco producers deny it, an important part of their promotions target on young audiences. The Health Promotion Unit at the North Western Regional Health Authority wished to combat the effects of tobacco advertising on the young. This was not so easy as it first appeared. Advertising agencies would not accept copy overtly attacking or parodying identifiable cigarette brands and even if they did, effective counter-advertising might, the RHA's legal advisers feared, expose them to claims for damages for loss of sales. The NWRHA's solution was to run a competition for under 16's to produce the best anti-smoking advertisement parodying a real cigarette advertisement. This avoided the risk of prosecution for damages because cigarettes cannot legally be sold to under 16's. Both the competition and the winning designs proved attractive news stories for local TV companies. Winning slogans and designs included 'There are Kings and there are Stupid Kings' (one king is smoking and coughing), 'Short Cut to the Tomb' (a sheet of silk, cut with a cross-shaped incision) and 'Dim' (in the appropriate livery and style).

promotion campaigns, for instance, have stimulated these responses from firms:

- Rationalizing the unhealthy behaviour or consumption (e.g. showing smoking as, say, a self-indulgent reward, as an aid to social poise and acceptability, or as a means to relax or concentrate) rather than disputing the health argument. A recent advertisement shows a suit-clad arm, hand and cigar above the slogan 'No decision I ever made couldn't wait half an hour'.
- Trying to shift debate onto matters more favourable to the firm or industry. Smoking, for example, is easier to defend as a civil liberty than in health terms.
- Claiming that 'We're not doctors', hence not competent to assess or comment upon medical evidence. This makes the firm appear deferential to the health professions and is taken as a licence to ignore the health promoters' views.
- Treating the health promotion campaign as a passing fad, presumably in the hope of making this a self-fulfilling prophecy. A recent poster announces 'Welcome back to butter'.
- Buying off the health organization with sponsorship. Peter Taylor reports the financial overtures made by certain British tobacco firms to the Health Education Council.[28]
- Creating or funding a front organization to counter NHS promotions on behalf of the firm or industry. FOREST is one example.[29]
- Sponsoring research to 'balance' or gainsay health promotions. Among other activities, for instance, the Office of Health Economics, which is extensively funded by pharmaceutical firms, includes in its publications

research (often of a high standard) arguing the therapeutic and economic benefits of pharmaceuticals.[30] Research is also used to try to anticipate or pre-empt, health promotions against dangerous products or industrial practices, for example by one of the major asbestos producers. Research is also undertaken to make the product actually safer, for instance in car design.

- Some firms respond by developing genuinely healthier products from their research e.g. low-alcohol drinks, low-dosage contraceptive tablets and low-fat foods.

The last two responses represent a qualified success for NHS promotional work and are arguably the most creditable responses that can be made by an organization against whom NHS social marketing or anti-marketing is directed.

Step 22. Select media and commission

Much as catering for the totality of patient needs or buyer demands requires a mix of products, meeting the diverse promotional objectives will require a mix of promotions.[31] The following list is not exhaustive but notes some practicalities of using the commoner media for NHS communications. Further advice can be obtained from the various handbooks on promotions.[32]

Printed material

Patient handbooks, leaflets and handouts e.g. 'mission statements', practice leaflets, newsletters can all be produced comparatively cheaply but to be persuasive and to attract readership must bear comparison with the mass of alternative reading material. They must be supplemented by materials for non-readers and the visually impaired. Posters are comparatively cheap but have many competitors, even when public or staff bother to read hospital notice boards. Roger Silver recommends the following guidelines in writing leaflets and similar copy.[33]

- Write short, jargon-free sentences.
- Assume that the reader has no previous knowledge.
- Be concise and check all facts.
- Where possible avoid text, logos, etc. which will date the material.
- Provide a contact name and phone number for the reader to find out more information.
- Say who published the material.

Video

Locally made videos are adequate for technical training and market research purposes. Cameras and editing equipment are now comparatively cheap. But videos used to deliver controversial or unfamiliar messages must compete with TV in terms of quality. These will almost certainly have to be bought in. In commissioning a video the choice of producer and director is critical (rather than the choice of company); seek one of the few with knowledge of health care, NHS, health policy and care groups. Vignette 5.6 describes one of the earliest NHS attempts. Computer graphics are currently fashionable but expensive (£5000 or more).

The press

Brad's and other directories of journalists are intended for advertisers primarily but do indicate what periodicals exist and their audiences.[34] News conferences and press releases are only one way of providing a service for journalists. Vignette 5.4 illustrates how database and information networking can also be used. In dealing with the press Silver recommends:[35]

- Take the initiative in offering stories.
- Meet their very tight deadlines.
- Never share an 'exclusive' story with a second reporter.
- Don't discriminate against particular journalists.
- Be accurate.

Vignette 5.6   More Like Ourselves

Exeter Health Authority set itself a target of providing community care for the majority of mentally-ill residents in Starcross Hospital during 1982–1985 and then closing that part of the hospital. Its strategy was to buy large houses in its rural catchment area, gain planning permission to convert these to community homes, convert them and then arrange for mentally-handicapped people from Starcross to move in. Three target audiences were identified whose co-operation was necessary: local planners, local residents who would become neighbours to mentally-handicapped people and some staff at Starcross Hospital itself. Staff in Exeter HA suspected that some residents still harboured mistaken and prejudicial views about mentally-handicapped people. In particular they wanted to correct any misapprehensions that mentally-handicapped people were dangerous to children, dirty or liable to 'lower the tone' of neighbourhoods.

To this end a promotional video entitled *More Like Ourselves* was produced for showing through public media such as shopping precinct video systems. The video explains what mental handicap is, comparing it to the more familiar physical disability, and introduces a number of mentally-handicapped people already in community care. They explain their everyday domestic activities, their hobbies and other pursuits and why they prefer living in the community to institutional care. For its time this video was an innovative and novel application of a marketing technique to health care. Some lessons have been learnt too; for example that videos for the public and for NHS staff require a different length of video and different methods of presentation. Since *More Like Ourselves* videos for these purposes have tended to be made at locality level rather than provided District wide.

- Try to anticipate difficult questions, especially about 'bad' news for the NHS organization.
- Never refuse a request for information.
- Give stories a 'human' touch if possible.
- Don't resent enquiries or be discouraged by the way the press angle and edit material.
- Don't attempt 'cover-ups'.

Published reports and books

These best suit specialist or political audiences. The impact can be increased if the report or book is launched with a press conference (as the Kings Fund do with some books and reports) but arranging access by journalists in national papers and periodicals is considerably easier in or near London.

'Events'

These range from open NHS meetings and hospital open days to royal visits, exhibitions and marathons. Whilst DHA and CHC meetings are (partly) public by law they are small use as a promotional medium; either the agenda is dry and remote from public interests, or the meeting can easily become a focus for political or pressure group activity. TV, local radio and journals are more likely to be attracted to events such as sports or royalty; as are the public. Competitions provide both interest and, if there is a prize, an incentive for assisting the NHS organization's objectives. Vignette 5.5 illustrates this point too.

Outreach to schools, workplaces or self-help groups

This can be achieved through the use of music, theatre, portable exhibitions, stand-up presentations and competitions. Music (live, recorded or taped) and theatre is especially useful for reaching young audiences, although commissioning material from well-known figures is likely to be difficult and expensive. Outreach to the CHC, organizations such as Age Concern and other consumer groups can be used to generate favourable comment from these comparatively objective parties, which may appear more convincing to the public than self-advertisement by the NHS itself.

Direct mail

This can be targeted and timed to the sponsor's choice but is expensive and, with junk mail burgeoning, often an unreliable way of informing an audience or of eliciting donations or volunteers.

Professional lobbyists

These can be hired to approach MPs and other influential figures on health policy matters. Often they are defeated parliamentary candidates, whose activity offers MPs a preliminary screening of supplicants.

Paid advertising

This is expensive and adverts for selling purposes tend to arouse more audience resistance than 'public service', political or charitable adverts. Paid advertising which has to be done anyway (e.g. to recruit staff) can also display the NHS organization's logo and a health slogan. Advertising competition for public attention is keen and there is a mass of secondary technical research on how to advertise effectively.[36] There is much to be said for buying in specialist advice on this (see below).

Logos, slogans and letterheads

These can be designed to reinforce a particular image of the NHS organization but as an aid to recognition or prompt to the memory they will have most effect if the slogan or logo is taken over into adverts, signs and other media. Give-away objects (pens, paper-weights, etc.) can be used for this but are often more useful in reminding staff of priorities than for external promotions.

Sponsorship

This can be used in two ways; NHS activity is often sponsored by non–NHS organizations (e.g. pharmaceutical firms) and non–NHS activities can be sponsored by NHS organizations (e.g. a DHA sponsoring a fun-run). Either way, the sponsor benefits by publicity and association with a popular organization or cause. However, this means that NHS organizations should be wary about which organizations they accept sponsorship from and on what terms. The HEA refused a sponsorship from the tobacco industry, both on principle and because a condition of the sponsorship was that the money was not to be used to investigate smoking-related disease.

Material incentives

These are a familiar commercial promotional method (e.g. 'reduced' prices, 'free' gifts, etc.). How much scope the internal market will leave for these in selling service contracts remains to be seen but individual hospital patients might, for instance, be offered the option of a private room or other 'extras' free of charge if they take up (say) cold surgery places at unpopular times. Cash incentives have to be decided in light of the NHS organization's overall costing and pricing policy; hence the NHS manager would do well to consult his or her finance department before offering them. Conferences and workshops are already used by pharmaceutical firms and private hospitals as a pretext for hospitality to potential buyers or referrers – material incentives in kind. There is a fine line between offering material incentives and bribing potential buyers; in this setting material incentives have to be offered or accepted strictly within NHS financial Standing Orders.

'Point of impact'

On NHS premises, these are the places at which users make their first contact with the NHS, such as medical records or porters' reception desks, switchboards, or GPs' receptionists. These might serve their communication purposes more effectively if they were remodelled as 'Patient Information Services' and telephone enquiry services.[37] Whilst their main task is to manage individual patients' enquiries and appointments, they can also be a focus for distributing other promotional materials.

Complaints procedures

These must, besides satisfying the regulatory and legal requirements and protecting NHS staff until any NHS fault is proved, give prompt feedback to the complainant (even if only a holding letter explaining how long it will take to give a proper answer) and, in the end, give the complainant good grounds for thinking that his or her complaint has been investigated thoroughly and any necessary remedy made (even if this is only an apology or an acknowledgement of the complainant's efforts in raising the issue).

Open information policy

Many NHS internal documents are dull even to their NHS readers but it is at least arguable that those which inform matters of public record (e.g. those informing public decisions at Health Authority meetings) can reasonably be made public and that the onus of proof should be placed on those who wish to deny the public access to NHS records (except records containing medically or commercially confidential information).

Word-of-mouth communication

This should not be under-estimated, so far as actual users of the NHS, their friends and relatives are concerned. It occurs inevitably and the informal networks are large. They work fast and free of charge. A patient discharged from hospital may within days have pronounced upon the experience to family, friends and GP. The only way for an NHS organization to exploit this promotional medium is to ensure that the patient's experience of the service meets or exceeds expectations. Hence two critical but often neglected promotional media are:

- Interaction between NHS staff, patients and the public is by far the most important element of patient experience and for conveying messages to NHS users. This implies a necessity both to communicate the current marketing strategies and their purposes to staff, and to train staff in interactive skills. The next chapter explains.
- Uniforms, the livery of buildings, equipment and vehicles, and the physical environment and ambience of NHS premises (its 'estate', in current jargon). These require professional design (by interior designers and architects not by engineers, clinicians or laundry managers) and periodic updating as fashions and tastes change, transforming the technical design concerns of the engineer, clinician, laundry manager, etc. into uniforms and estate which are attractive to patients and staff and boost their confidence besides being technically efficient.

The delivey of an NHS service has therefore to be designed with promotional, and other, considerations in mind. Chapter 6 explains.

In choosing promotional media and materials it is necessary to consider the following questions:

- What is the purpose of each promotional medium – to raise awareness? to change health behaviours? to shift patterns of service uptake or referral patterns? to change the public image of a client group? to educate about a particular disease? Only if this is clear can the effectiveness of the promotion be defined and tracked.
- How each promotional medium is to be used; for instance whether the target audience will be able to give the medium their undivided attention or whether it will be competing with other adverts, signs, background noise, etc. Will the promotional material be delivered by NHS staff, by a professional trainer or educator, by friends or relatives, or selected by the patient himself?
- Communicational effectiveness. It is important to evaluate the effectiveness of promotional materials; some promotional activities not merely fail but actually discredit the intended message.[38] New promotional materials should be pilot tested on a small sample of the target audience to assess whether they produce recognition, understanding, recall or behavioural change. The cycle of inventing, pilot testing, evaluating, adapting and testing again until a satisfactory promotion is developed is analogous to steps E and F in the market research process described in Chapter 4.
- Reaching the target audiences. Different media are likely to appeal to, and to influence, each target audience. (Densely written materials are most likely to appeal to educated populations; Welsh language materials may be desirable for Welsh-speakers etc.).
- The 'promotional mix'. Just as service quality specifications may have to differ for different user segments so may the promotional messages and media. This creates a need to check the consistency of messages, logos, etc. across the different media and targets, and between internal and external communications, so that the different promotional materials become

mutually reinforcing instead of undermining each other.[39] External messages must be consistent with internal messages and reward policy and may include project publicity (step 20) and the marketer's implementation method itself (step 19) e.g. publicizing the work of PSTs.

- Timing. Some promotional activities can be timed to coincide closely with service changes (e.g. TV adverts) or to reinforce a message by repetition. Repetition is less simple to manage than it seems. The effect of the promotional medium in generating recall and response 'wears out' over some weeks after the audience are exposed. But it is only wise to repeat the promotion if its effects were positive; otherwise repetition actually subverts the intended message.[40] Hence one should track the effects of the first promotional wave before repeating it.

- Cost. Promotional materials are not cheap. Expect to pay say £40 000 for a professionally-designed logo and substantial brochure (including the cost of the first print runs). Professionally made videos cost £1000–£1500 per finished minute plus computer graphics, specially commissioned music, etc. A mailshot may cost over £10 000, a one-page advert in a national paper £20 000 or more. A professional lobbyist costs in the range £150 –£600 per day. A standard way of comparing the cost of different mass media is by the price per 1000 of the target audience reached or per response generated or (for sellers) by a straightforward cost–benefit analysis.

- Ethical considerations. The confidentiality of patient information, the restrictions on publicity imposed by the BMA ethical code and its equivalents in other professions and the fact that the borderline between material incentives and bribery is sometimes indistinct.

Promotional work, like market research, is in certain conditions better carried out by an external contractor than within the NHS. This is especially likely when the promotional material has to compete with other organizations' promotions and messages. Here 'creative', design and presentation expertise of a comparable standard is required and at present this expertise is very scarce in the NHS. An external provider is also required when a fresh and critical re-working of outdated promotional material is required, e.g. to update staff uniforms or interior design. Small NHS organizations such as general practices will not find it practicable to set up a permanent promotional staff and will therefore have to buy promotional materials *ad hoc*. The brief for an external provider of promotion work should be analogous to the brief for an external market researcher (see Chapter 3), stating the target audiences, the behavioural or attitudinal objectives and the main messages. Check who owns copyright (if you intend to use logos, photos, etc. for several purposes) and demand the right to see and alter or veto copy before it is used. Possible consultancies can be found through exhibitions, directories, marketing and media journals (e.g. *Marketing, Campaign*) or by recommendation through other NHS bodies or education centres. Promotional work carried out within an NHS organization is probably best provided by a specialized wing of the marketing function; Chapter 6 explains this too.

Chapter 6

Service design and tracking

Whilst the communications strategy is being implemented the design and actual delivery of services has to occur (and be co-ordinated with the promotional work). This chapter explains the steps involved, following the right-hand branch from step 17 in Figure 5.1. The NHS internal market makes these steps primarily applicable to the provider organizations, and the scale of marketing activity they presuppose will be found in hospitals and similar-sized organizations rather than any but the largest general practices.

Service design and organization

Step 18B. Service design

Service design is mainly the concern of the NHS provider, as it is the process for deciding the practical means to realize the quality specification agreed with the provider as a corollary of the service contract (steps 10, 15). The essence of the task is to design the service to meet buyer demands (in the case of sellers) or user needs (in the case of DMUs). A service design is therefore more than an operational policy in its standard NHS form, which does little more than stipulate the occupational division of labour within a hospital or general practice (for instance by stating whether reception desks will be staffed by porters, secretaries or medical records workers). The service design specifies what Donabedian calls the 'structure' and (part of) the 'process' of care, just as the quality specification specifies (the rest of) 'process' and 'outcome'.[1] A distinctive service design can powerfully differentiate a health service provider. For instance, the techniques of simple cold surgery are often much the same wherever performed. If a provider is to gain a competitive advantage in such services it is precisely in such matters as presentation of services, its staff's reputation for helpfulness, the availability of surgery at times to suit the patient and so on.

The more radical approach to service design draws on the results of health service research and development (see step 11). Ideas for service design can be drawn from two sources. Examination of 'good practice', competitor and substitute services, and methods and sources for this has already been mentioned (pp. 67f. and pp. 90f.) in explaining how to produce a service quality specification. A second source is applied research and development work initiated within the NHS organization. This tends to be initiated by interested individual clinicians and managers, or more rarely, sponsored in a unit or general practice by RHAs, the Department of Health, the NHSTA or foundations such as the Nuffield Provincial Hospitals Trust. In practice the second source will be more episodic and patchy because the NHS almost entirely lacks any overall research and development strategy. One task for the marketing or quality assurance manager is therefore to keep abreast of such activities in his or her own NHS organization and of their potential service applications. For service design purposes, these sources have to be studied not only for the outcomes and iatrogenesis reported but to reveal the human, physical, information, organizational, communications and other inputs that 'good practice' requires. The purpose is to describe the new quality chain required to implement the service.

A less radical (but often more practicable) approach is to redesign the existing quality chain (step 7). This is done by itemizing the human resources, physical facilities and care activities necessary at each stage of the quality chain, describing these inputs and activities in terms of the user's experience. A comprehensive operational policy of the traditional NHS kind – if it exists – will already identify the activities and facilities necessary to consider in producing a service design.

Which approach is more appropriate depends upon what stage of its 'product life cycle' the existing service design is at. Figure 1.1 illustrated the main stages in the product life cycle. In health service terms, the innovation stage consists of perfecting the new service technically, making it effective, safe and ethically acceptable through limited, experimental use in only a few locations (e.g. *in utero* fetal surgery, in 1990). The dissemination stage sees the spread of the service to most Regions, then to most Districts (e.g. heart transplants). A mature service is generally available (e.g. day surgery for minor cold work). Obsolescence sets in when a new service design enters its dissemination stage and supersedes the existing form of service (e.g. endos-copy or lithotrity replacing the surgical removal of gallstones). For a service at the innovation and obsolescent stages the radical approach to service design is likely to be more applicable, while quality chain redesign will be more applicable at the dissemination and mature stages.

When available, accreditation will assist both approaches to service design. Australian and US accreditation systems (from which an NHS accreditation system is unlikely to differ radically in its early days) not only enumerate systematically the main productive activities making up a health service but set standards for these activities, their management and record-ing. Meanwhile the Australian and US accreditation manuals are worth consulting as a surrogate. (However these manuals are difficult to obtain except directly from the respective accreditation organizations and the US manual is expensive: some $500.)

The purpose of either approach is to stipulate how each input is to be selected or provided, and how the inputs are combined, concentrating on two aspects of each activity or facility:

- Functional aspect – the way in which the service meets its central objectives (whether commercial or 'real' health objectives). The technical specification of the process of care is central to this – methods of treatment, diagnostic and paramedical services, safety measures, etc. Organizational characteristics such as referral, booking and discharge procedures or medical records systems are also 'functional' aspects. The functional aspect of service design should above all be guided by the technical experts (clinical staff, medical records, engineers, etc.). On clinical matters the medical directors and paramedical managers are the obvious source or channel for this. It is important to set functional standards high enough. A 97% success rate for each procedure in a treatment plan sounds a high standard; but if a patient's treatment plan is for five procedures in sequence the probability of the whole episode being provided to standard is only $0.97^5 = 86\%$. A patient on a course of 22 such procedures has less than a 50% chance of getting fully up-to-standard care. (If 'procedures' are taken to include tests, 22 procedures is not many for an in-patient episode.)[2]
- Semiotic aspect – the way in which the physical facilities and events in the quality chain also have a promotional effect (see Chapter 5) because users and staff interpret, or use, these characteristics as social signs. For instance a three hour wait for a three minute consultation might reasonably be taken as a sign that the hospital implicitly values the consultant's time sixty times as much as the patient's. Prompt and courteous treatment gives an opposite impression. Staff also interpret facilities and events in this way.

The distinction between 'functional' and 'semiotic' aspects is not the same as the provider-led : user-led demarcation. The semiotic aspects of the service are, in the terminology explained at step 8, 'rationally user-led' because what is relevant to the semiotic aspects of service design is how the user interprets the promotional 'signs' of staff attitude and manner, uniforms, the appearance of buildings, etc. (For these purposes NHS staff can be regarded as one category of 'user'.) These aspects of service design can be 'read off' from market research results. Some of the functional aspects are also user-led (e.g. how non-ambulance transport to and from hospital is organized), some provider-led (e.g. clinical policy on radical mastectomy). The former are also read off from market research, the latter from evaluations and market research into competing services (see pp. 67–8).

Neither is the distinction between 'functional' and 'semiotic' aspects of the service the same as the clinical : non-clinical demarcation. It is necessary to ensure that the semiotic aspects of clinical care are consciously designed (e.g. to decide whether doctors will introduce themselves and explain the purpose of the consultation, whether they will give the patient opportunity to choose between alternative treatment plans where available, etc.). It is equally necessary to design the functional aspects of non-clinical services (e.g. how to decide how fast it must be possible to empty the building if there is a fire, or to decide what information the receptionist must succeed in communicating to incoming patients). Semiotic aspects of the service, such as building design or the degree of freedom patients have in the activities of daily life, can have therapeutic or iatrogenic effects (above all, institutionalization[3]) especially in long-term care and have to be designed with this in mind. The resulting service design consists of a set of specifications for the process of care (for example; 'All patients will be spoken to by a member of staff and taken for triage within one minute of arrival at A&E' or 'Vegetarian meals, a "healthy eating" meal and a meal acceptable to Moslems and Jews will be available on every menu'). Chapter 3 explained how the quality chain itself is reconstructed empirically using market research. It also explained how market research can be used to specify user-led characteristics of the service, and evaluations and competitor analyses to specify the provider-led characteristics. Analogously, market research results can be used to determine the user-led standards of service design. Service characteristics can be 'read off' directly from market research findings such as that certain groups of elderly people tend to value having a telephone much more than having a television, are more prone than younger people to discuss non-medical matters with their GP[4] and want chiropody, help with bathing, domestic chores and mobility.[5] Accreditation, evaluation and competitor analysis can be used to determine the provider-led aspects of service design; sources for this data are as described on p. 90.

In practice different service design requirements may conflict. Sometimes managers will confront straightforward trade-offs (e.g. between a long wait before tests and consultation begin and a long wait between the test and the consultation). If functional and semiotic requirements conflict, it will ordinarily be necessary to give functional requirements priority over the semiotic (e.g. operating theatre staff cannot, in interests of patient safety, usually wear their 'normal' clothes). However the conflict may also indicate the need for further research and development (e.g. to find out how the ordinary furnishings necessary to give a home-like ambience to a long-stay ward can also be made sufficiently durable and fire-proof). Table 6.1 outlines part of a fictional service design for the quality chain illustrated at Figure 3.3.

Before the full-scale introduction of a new service design marketers recommend that the proposal be screened for consistency with other health service objectives in much the same way as a quality specification is (see step 11, p. 73). If it survives, the proposal should next undergo 'concept testing', i.e. the use of market research to check whether buyers and users are likely to find the concept of the new service acceptable in principle. Users will accept a new product with obvious limitations provided it offers over-compensating benefits.[6] After this, a draft business and a marketing strategy can be produced for the new service, to ensure that it will be viable commercially and in marketing terms. If the proposal survives these checks, the next task is a trial of a pilot version.[7] The latter is especially necessary when new clinical techniques are being included in the service design. Practical considerations in relating clinical trials to service design include:

Table 6.1 Part of a fictional service design for hospital services for the part quality chain shown in Figure 3.3

Quality chain event	Functional specification	Semiotic specification
Offer of appointment	Written offer to be sent within 7 days of GP referral. Offer exact appointment time. Chase up non-replies after 14 days	Personalized top copy letter on headed paper, enclosing introductory leaflet on the hospital
Wait to visit OPD	No wait to exceed 12 weeks from GP referral	Update letter in above format sent to patient every 4 weeks explaining wait, apologizing and confirming appointment still booked
Hospital transport service	Patients to reach hospital not more than 15 minutes before and not later than 5 minutes after appointment time	Clean modern vehicle with DHA livery or official badge, uniformed driver when DHA employee
Reaching reception	Signs legible from 25 metres by people with normal vision. Signs at all public entrances to site and building, and at all corridor junctions inside building	Clean signs in DHA colours and with DHA logo. Text in English and Welsh
Reception	No queue longer than 5 persons or 5 minutes. Desk staffed continuously from 0800 to 1730 Monday to Saturday	All patients to be addressed by name. Tidy display of notices and publications (no DIY signs taped on the walls). Receptionist to explain arrangement for any preliminary tests
Decision on preliminary tests	To be made by consultant before appointment on basis of referral note and any previous medical record	Test to be explained to patient in private by member of staff administering it
Wait for tests	95% of patients to wait less than 30 minutes for results	Staff to explain delay if wait exceeds 30 minutes
Medical consultation	All patients to be seen by consultant at least once during episode	Doctors to introduce selves, and anyone else present. Permission always to be asked for presence of students. Patients to have opportunity to question or amend treatment plan

- Ensuring that an ethical committee system exists or can be constructed to review the trial protocols before evaluation begins. Although this is indispensable for safeguarding patients, health care ethicists or staff with a training in health care ethics can probably give a more penetrating assessment of the ethical implications of new clinical techniques in morally complex or subtle areas of care such as reproductive technologies (IVF, etc.) and terminal care. The NHS manager can also consult a burgeoning literature on these matters.[8]
- Checking that patients participating give informed consent. It is always good research practice to ensure that explanations of the trial are given and patient consent sought by staff without any (other) interest in the trial or its results.
- Informing oneself of at least the principles and methods of evaluation[9] so as to be able to judge if the trial was well-constructed and how valid the results are likely to be. Remember, however, that even the paradigm of scientifically reputable evaluation, the randomized control trial with double-blind and crossover, can sometimes yield faulty results.[10] Hence also get a technically informed second (and independent) opinion on the substantive results of the trial before deciding whether to incorporate the innovation into a service design.
- Checking the financial implications of trials, both in terms of revenue and capital costs and to ensure that the proceeds of any sponsorship from pharmaceutical or other firms actually find their way into NHS funds.

Experiments and pilots also enable comparatively minor design and implementation problems to be identified and remedied at the outset. Table 4.1 (p. 83) outlines the market research approach required. Many texts and a few journals (e.g. the *International Journal of Technology Assessment in Health Care*, the *Journal of Health Economics*) are available to demonstrate evaluative methods and report results of recent evaluations.

Step 19B. Organize management of the marketing aspects

There are at least five ways in which NHS providers can organize themselves internally to implement the service design and the marketing activity which supports it.

Conventional line management (which is not restricted to DMUs nor the only way a DMU can implement a service design) is one. In this case the processes of business planning, service specification, the award of service contract and service design supersede the received NHS service planning methods developed since 1974 ('supersede', not 'replace', because many of the characteristics of the 1974 system such as the epidemiological input, have a place in the activities described above). The resulting objectives, specifications and service design are then implemented by being transmitted downwards, and their achievement monitored, through the existing IPR, performance related pay, contract renewal procedures, annual review and general management hierarchies with the usual consultations with the medical establishment, trade unions and other centres of power. What marketing adds to NHS management in this case is not so much new managerial structures (except for the marketing infrastructure described below) but a new content and new priorities for existing NHS management. Many other activities are also implemented in this way, however, so implementing a marketing strategy through line management requires strong general manager commitment to marketing and leadership; more on this below. The line management structure should enable a single manager to be identified as responsible for each quality chain.

Quality circles supplementing existing line management is a second method. (Quality circles take various names in the NHS e.g. 'Personal Service Teams', 'Patient Care Groups'.) Quality circles consist of volunteers who meet regularly to discuss service delivery and ways to improve it, often on the basis of their own market research, and attempt to implement the proposals they generate. In effect, they operate a condensed informal version of the whole marketing process. Quality circles are suitable for general practices besides hospitals. However, NHS organizations have mixed success with them in practice. Conditions favouring success for quality circles include:[11]

- Low staff turnover, since quality circles draw on informal networks.
- Fairly high staff morale.
- A clear remit stating areas where the quality circle has discretion and those (e.g. industrial relations policy) which are not their concern.
- Starting with a pilot scheme, but one large enough to absorb a small number of failures.
- Demonstrable independence of line management. The UGM and other line managers must be willing to take the 'risk' of 'letting go' of close control, intervening only to offer resource support or prevent a crisis. But also;
- Senior managers' support for the quality circles. It is necessary to explain the purpose and working of quality circles to middle managers, especially those in clinical professions, so that they support the quality circles rather than ignore or obstruct them because they feel bypassed or threatened.
- Finding an organizational means of co-ordinating quality circles in many parts of a hospital with the line management. Vignette 6.1 shows how one unit addressed this.
- Participants' ability to set aside distinctions of rank, status and occupation within quality circle meetings. One nurse manager found that members of the ward quality circle still deferred to her in quality circle meetings. She solved this problem by giving the other members chairs but sitting on the floor herself.
- Being able to demonstrate some successes in the early days and then perhaps six months later to maintain momentum once initial enthusiasm has flagged.

Vignette 6.1   Quality circles and line management

As the quality management strategy at Stafford DGH took shape during 1989, the question arose of how to extend the Quality Management Groups (comparable to quality circles) from their point of origin in the out-patient's department across the whole hospital and how to integrate them with the existing team briefing system. This also raised the question of how to relate the Quality Management Groups to each other, to the existing management structure and to other quality management initiatives in the District. The solution chosen is shown in Figure 6.1 below (an asterisk indicates that the briefing team has one member who is also a member of the UMT and of the Quality Steering Group).

- Pilot experimentally first to learn practically how to do, get positive models for success and show results.
- Train leaders in chairmanship and communicate the results of the group's work to line managers.
- Train facilitators in the informal social processes of quality circles and how to organize workload.
- Publicize and reward success.

   Internal marketing (the third method) is undertaken by setting up marketing interfaces within the NHS organization, so that departments who may have few dealings with patients or public treat as their 'customer' the staff who do. For example an estates department would then identify other wards and departments as the 'customers' for its building and decorating work, consultants, laboratories, CSSD, etc. as the 'customer' for electrical and mechanical repairs and so on. The department then conducts market research into these 'customers'' service requirements and modifies its own activities accordingly. In short, the department reproduces, in simplified form, the marketing cycle described here. Internal marketing can be combined with orthodox line management or quality circles. Software packages and techniques such as 'performance mapping' and 'Q-mapping' are commercially available to provide a planning framework for the process.

   Quality Improvement Teams (fourthly) are project teams or 'task forces' briefed to investigate a particular quality or marketing issue, often through the QIT's own market research, and implement action. They are responsible to the line manager for a department, ward or other service but their membership cuts across the formal organizational demarcations of occupation and line management. This enables them to form a more rounded view of the quality chain and service design than conventional NHS management structures usually allow at middle or supervisory level. These teams may be permanent or have a life limited to a single task. The main condition of success is that the members have sufficient power in the departments or wards constituting the service to enable the QIT to take and implement

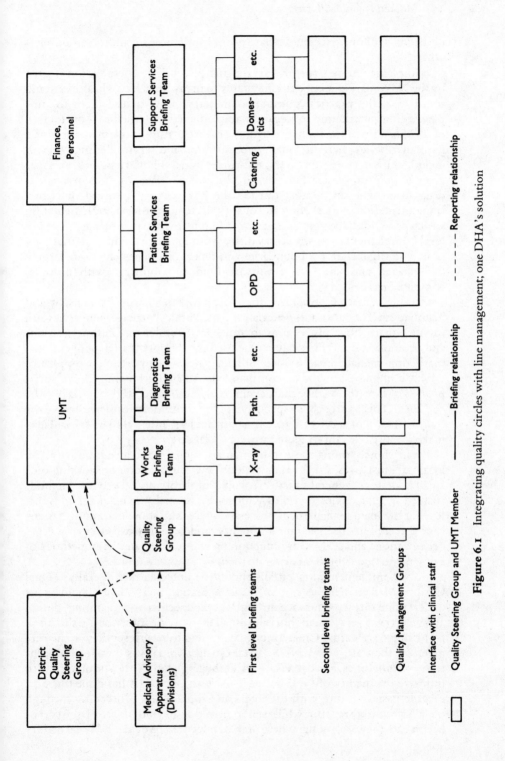

Figure 6.1 Integrating quality circles with line management; one DHA's solution

decisions without excessive delays for consultation or authorization elsewhere.

Implementation structures are the fifth possibility. These are not created by the NHS marketer but exist inevitably in many branches of health care and social care; the practical question is therefore how to use them for implementing a marketing strategy. An implementation structure is the totality of all those involved (either assisting or obstructing) implementation of a particular policy; here the quality specification and service design.[12] It will include statutory services, users, informal carers, voluntary bodies, pressure groups, political bodies and even (in the case of services to groups such as drug users who are almost outside the law) people involved in crime. Implementation of marketing and quality strategies through implementation structures tends to be very decentralized (often down to care manager and GP level). Implementation structures differ from line management in that they transcend organizational boundaries and managerial hierarchies, are largely self-selected and undesigned and are fluid and informal with mutiple, complex linkages.[13]

Implementation structures therefore work primarily by consent and negotiation. The more authoritarian and hierarchical management styles still found in many NHS professions are much less useful here. Communications and promotional activities have to be used much more than in conventional marketing management to win other agencies' support and compliance which cannot be bought or commanded. An understanding of the social process of care (the quality chain again) is especially necessary but likely to be complex. This approach is especially apt for community care because of the fragmentation of services across many providers. Internal markets will also make it more relevant to acute care and social care.

The choice among these implementation methods depends above all on local circumstances. NHS organizations new to marketing or working on a small scale (e.g. general practices) would probably do best to use methods such as quality circles or QITs which are essentially managerial add-ons, leaving the main management processes intact until some marketing experience and skill has been acquired. Quality circles already exist in many NHS organizations and if these are functioning successfully any new methods of implementation should incorporate them.

Two implementation pitfalls should be noted. Taken literally, 'Total Quality Management' is not an implementation method. It would mean undertaking quality assurance throughout the specification, planning, design and delivery of services; in short almost all the activities described in this book from step 6 onwards. Chief among the inputs to health services is the care given by the staff. Many NHS 'Total Quality' initiatives therefore concentrate – sometimes exclusively – on enthusing staff with a motivation to improve the quality of NHS services. At least one DHA has done this on a cascade basis, starting with managers and trainers and proceeding through the whole workforce. But whilst staff motivation and morale are a large part of health care they are not the whole of it, as may now be evident. 'Total quality management' in the sense of re-motivating staff is one of the forms of internal communication described below. Secondly, avoid steering committees as a vehicle for implementation (except perhaps when they really are for steering and co-ordinating multiple marketing projects). The usual NHS committee processes of debate, consultation and consensus are laboriously slow at best, and likely to be an especially slow and laborious means of implementing unfamiliar and controversial work such as NHS marketing.

Sooner or later, however, NHS line management must be used to implement marketing strategy if marketing and quality assurance are to be more than occasional, marginal extras in NHS activity. This raises the question of how a marketing function can be created and how it should be organized.

The use of marketing activities as a support to NHS clinicians and line managers has been emphasized, and the scarcity of marketing resources in the NHS often noted. So the optimal way to organize an NHS marketing function is as a staff function reporting to the general manager (or equivalent) but from which other line managers and clinicians could also commission work *ad hoc*. The marketing function would then function primarily through internal marketing to these clients, similar to the way NHS finance departments are intended to work. Since the internal market will create conflicts of commercial interests between buyers and sellers and among sellers, and since in directly managed NHS services the District and the Unit levels have different foci of marketing interests, each NHS organization will require its own marketing function.

A comprehensive (but not over-comprehensive) marketing department in an NHS organization would therefore:

- Provide marketing inputs and assessments for NHS business planning (requires liaison with the finance function and, in DHAs, the directorate of public health).
- Provide technical advice on market research design and execution.
- Conduct market research and technical evaluations, either through its own staff or;
- Select, brief, commission and control external providers of market research or evaluation.
- Maintain (or provide access to) databases on past evaluations, market research, clinical trials and tracking information.
- Ensure that clinical audit develops and feed the summary results into marketing, quality assurance and general management activities as described in Chapters 3–6.
- Analyse and present market research results.
- Provide technical advice on the semiotic aspects of service design, and access sources of advice on the functional aspect. This will require liaison with, or even the recruitment of, clinicians and epidemiologists.
- Identify research and development tasks and test experimental new services.

- Assist health promoters, health educators and intersectoral planners in selecting and developing their communications.
- Design and implement communications strategies on health policy and for image-building (or commission outside suppliers to do so).
- Train staff in marketing, quality assurance, communication and related matters (see below).
- Assist the design of medical records and other information systems to ensure these contribute to marketing work and quality assurance.

It bears repeating that this is to be done as an aid to the direct management of the service; hence on the line manager's behalf. The marketing or quality assurance manager would therefore ideally be deputy to the general manager, especially in provider organizations. Obviously the marketing function would have different emphases and size in different NHS organizations. However few if any NHS organizations are yet able to sustain a marketing function of this complexity. So meanwhile the key elements in the role for existing NHS quality assurance co-ordinators include:

- Assisting line managers and clinicians in initiating and implementing the steps described in Chapters 3–6.
- Developing the marketing function with the form and activities noted above, including developing and updating the knowledge and skills of the QA co-ordinator and his or her staff. This can be done through conferences, formal education and training, and membership of marketing, quality assurance and market research organizations (e.g. NAQA, the Marketing Society). Some marketing organizations (e.g. the Marketing Society) restrict membership to practising marketers but in the internal market NHS quality assurance and marketing managers will increasingly become exactly this.
- The internal marketing of marketing, quality assurance and communications to general managers, department heads, clinicians and other managers.

Service delivery

Step 20B. Leadership, rewards and internal communications

Leadership from step 1 has much the same necessity in marketing as in other managerial activities but its role becomes most apparent when the focus of marketing activity moves outside the comparatively specialized areas of market research, service design, etc. to changing the working practices of large numbers of NHS staff. This is achieved by getting high-status or powerful figures to support the marketing strategy actively and conspicuously, through internal communications and through rewards.

The leading figures whose active support the marketer must, in practice, win are firstly the Health Authority itself, particularly the chairman or woman. General Managers' support is equally necessary, especially if they intend to delegate most of the detailed marketing work to a quality assurance manager or other subordinate. Doctors inevitably play a leading role not only because of their *de facto* power in influencing resource use and whether new service designs can be implemented in the critical, clinical areas, but because the medical profession is the role model which most other clinical professions in the NHS aspire to imitate. Heads of other clinical professions can set a stamp of professional credibility on the marketing work and to prevent professional considerations being cited to legitimate indifference or obstruction. (This is not to deny the duty of the professional head to defend professional considerations against marketing considerations when there really is a conflict; an increasingly likely prospect in the more commercialized areas of NHS work.) Informal leaders are individual enthusiasts for marketing or quality assurance at ward or department level. These are often overlooked but they are critical to ensuring that service design is implemented, and reviewed critical, through to the bedside or workbench.

The support required consists of:

- Giving marketing activity a guaranteed and a high place on managerial agendas and in the IPR and review processes.
- Publicly reporting and endorsing marketing successes.
- Guaranteeing the cash and other resources required for the marketing activities (see below).
- Putting the leaders' personal influence behind the marketing activity in negotiations with doctors, trade unions and other power centres.
- 'Figurehead' activities (e.g. turning up at induction or training days to show personal support for current marketing activity).
- Modelling the behaviours expected of other staff. This includes being seen to give marketing activity much time, attention and importance and by demonstrating by one's own practice how staff are expected to speak to patients, deal with complaints and enquiries, etc.

A frequently-encountered problem is how to maintain interest in a marketing initiative after the first six months when the initial enthusiasm wears off. Besides continuing the above support after the initial period, the manager responsible for the marketing activity can:

- Arrange for tracking data showing the impact of the activity to become available towards the end of the first six months and regularly thereafter.
- Provide extra resources or other rewards then.
- Where possible, arrange for the resulting service changes to be permanently incorporated into the 'normal' management and working practice, so that the resulting service changes cannot be dismissed as temporary, marginal 'pilots' or 'experiments', having let staff know at the outset that this may occur.
- Recruit staff who contributed during the first six months to help with

spreading the activities they have invented elsewhere in the DHA, unit or practice.
- Set up permanent internal communications systems to report good practice and marketing successes, especially any tangible benefits to patients and staff.

The task of internal communications for the purpose of implementing a service design is to let staff know what problems have arisen with existing services, how NHS staff can contribute to improving matters, and the benefits to be expected. The essence of successful communication is, so far as practicable, to let staff arrive by their own thinking at the ideas which support the redesign of services, different attitudes to patients, etc. The most effective media for communicating the proposed service changes and the reasons for them are therefore interactive media such as staff training events, team briefings, quality circles and staff meetings. (These are, however, more demanding of managers' time and interactive skills than printed materials or video.) Communication consultancies are willing to undertake this work for NHS managers acting, in the words of one,[14] as an 'internal sales force'. Many of the so-called 'Total Quality Management' programmes (and handbooks[15]) tend to concentrate on this aspect of internal communications.

Internal communication for marketing purposes becomes easier if staff have been kept informed from step 1 what marketing activities will occur and why, have contributed to market research and been presented with the results. This recommends a comparatively open style of management in marketing matters. One way to identify messages for communication internally is to compare staff attitudes and beliefs about the service with those (and other market research and evaluative data) about patients' experiences. The largest gaps show main communication tasks (e.g. if staff imagine that most patients do not want to understand how the treatment works but patients express a different view) and the data themselves offer a comparatively objective way of showing staff where changes in the service in personal behaviour may be necessary. Messages for internal communication have to be consistent with those for external consumption, because NHS staff will also see any TV adverts, leaflets, etc. aimed at users and the public. Promotional materials must also bear comparison, in terms of presentation and quality, with those used externally; otherwise staff are entitled to conclude that management care less about communication with them than about patients, public or buyers. (The same applies to the quality of furnishings, food, etc. supplied to staff.)

Reward policy can also be used to implement marketing changes in services. However it is salutary for NHS managers to compare the activities and personal attributes that NHS pay and conditions actually reward, with those specified by the service design. NHS managers at or below middle level have little discretion for giving or withholding these rewards but some non-cash incentives will often lie within their gift. Praise for success is one. One northern children's ward used to run a 'Doctor of the Week' noticeboard on which the children who were able wrote up an article (with pictures to illustrate!) about the doctor whose work had most captured their imagination during the week. (Why should this sort of recognition be restricted to doctors?) Opportunity for training, education and development, whether in form of job rotation, formal training events or study leave can also be used.

Step 21B. Resourcing

Because marketing activities have until recently been marginal to NHS activities, NHS managers can easily take too narrow a view of the resources required. These comprise not only the marginal resources for market research, internal communications (see above), modification to buildings, etc. Service design implies a review of the whole range of resources required to deliver a service. Resourcing the marketing activity therefore requires attention to staffing, the NHS estate, and purchasing.

Staffing

Most NHS service designs will emphasize the personal aspects of care provided by staff. Many of the personal characteristics which make a member of staff good at this (e.g. general intelligence, patience, ability to listen, self-presentation) will largely be determined by the time the individual reaches working age. Staff recruitment and selection is therefore a critical means of implementing a service design, and it falls to line managers to ensure that job specifications, person specifications, recruitment advertisements, and selection criteria give weight to the personal characteristics required for implementing the service design besides the more obvious technical qualifications, professional registration, etc. (Obviously this will be harder to achieve with scarce staff groups such as speech therapists.) One way to do this is to use the service quality specification and service design as a direct source for writing job descriptions and IPR agendas. Similar considerations apply to day-to-day decisions about deployment of existing staff and setting of personal objectives through IPR. They apply to clinicians as well as non-clinical staff. The market research required to support staff recruitment is mentioned in Table 3.5 and the promotional uses of staff recruitment campaigns in Chapter 5. Chapter 3 notes the types of training in NHS marketing appropriate to different categories of staff.

NHS estates

These require design not only for professional convenience and ease of maintenance but above all as the place in which the designed service can be delivered. This requires attention to such aspects of building design as privacy for patients, a domestic scale of buildings for long-term care, capacity to avoid potential bottlenecks at peak periods in busy clinics and a layout intelligible to patients and public. For these purposes the estates service must provide (or commission) interior design services. Organizations such as Arts for Health can provide practical help in these matters. There is a small but growing research interest in the possibility that building design and ambiences has a measurable therapeutic effect. This is still under research but it is necessary for estates managers also to keep abreast of these developments. For these purposes the optimal relation between the estates function and line manager may be an internal marketing relation (see above), but this is not to rule out estates managers conducting their own market research into patients' and public preferences for health building design, decoration and signposting (or including such questions in the line managers' market research).

Purchasing

The 'supplies' function is subject to similar considerations. A supplies department can conduct its own market research on patients, public and staff to discover which sorts of furnishings, teabags, etc. they ordinarily prefer and why. Taking tea, for instance, is as much a social occasion and a psychological comfort for patients as a way of taking hot liquids in a form cheap and convenient to the NHS.

Cash

Cash is required for all this. There is no reason to believe that higher quality health services are cheaper in the short run; if anything the opposite is likely to be the case because marketed health services care will probably include additional activities and higher quality (often costlier) inputs. In conventional markets higher value-added products tend to increase profits but there is no reason to expect *a priori* that NHS internal markets will work this way. The most visible cash cost of a service redesign is the initial investment to develop the redesigned service to the point where it becomes possible to provide the service as a directly-managed service or to seek service contracts for it.

NHS sellers will soon face the risk (novel to them) of their capital spending having nothing to show for it. Launching new commercial services is inherently risky with a high failure rate during the first year. The risk can be minimized by considering the following points when deciding how much capital to venture on developing a new form of service (they also apply to secondary 'income generating' activities).

- How much can the organization afford to invest? This also places a ceiling on the amount of income that sellers can make from the redesigned service in the internal market. New SGT services are likely to require working capital for wages, equipment and consumables until cash flow begins.
- What range of outcomes is possible for each income-generating option in the worst event, in the best event, and in the most probable event?[16] The worst event is lowest *guaranteed* income, which may be nothing or even a

loss, minus the investment mentioned above. (If accounting systems allow it, these incomes may be discounted for time and for probability.) Any option whose worst event exceeds what the NHS seller can afford to lose should be rejected. The risk-minimizing decision follows a 'maximin' rule: select the option, whose worst possible result (i.e. whose guaranteed return) is highest. (This may differ from the option whose likeliest or whose best return is highest.)

- If it fails, at what point would the redesigned service be discontinued? If this point is defined in cash terms, a ceiling is placed on the seller's possible financial loss. This decision identifies a critical financial tracking variable and its trigger point.

Tracking

Step 22. Select tracking variables and periodicity

Tracking is the application of market research to the evaluation and monitoring of services against their quality specification, service contract requirements and service design. It enables an NHS organization to learn from its practical experience how to conduct its marketing activities, how to revise and raise its service quality specifications and improve its promotional activity. Its practical importance is therefore hard to understate. The preliminary to tracking is to select what variables to track, the reporting relations and the periodicity of tracking.

Tracking variables

Tracking variables are selected from the business plan (see step 6), the service quality specification (step 10), the service contract (step 15), the communications objectives (step 18A and the service design (step 18B), plus any legal or information requirements ('feeding the beast', in current NHS jargon) imposed by the RHA, NHS Management Executive or central government. Two kinds of tracking variable are required for NHS purposes. The more obvious is to monitor the effects of NHS marketing activity in terms of service utilization, outcome, iatrogenesis, return to the community, etc. Less obvious, but no less important both for health promotion and for future business planning in internal markets, is to monitor how political opponents and competitors, respectively, respond to the effects of the NHS organization's marketing. The main criteria for selecting tracking variables are:

- Centrality to the business plan (e.g. mortality rates for preventable or treatable disease for a DHA, profit rate for an SGT).
- Centrality to the service contract, especially those which may trigger extra rewards or penalties (e.g. delays in sending GPs' post-discharge reports on their patients referred to the hospital).

- Aspects of services or communication which are critical to achieving the two above (e.g. the ability of an SGT hospital with a per-case or a cost-and-volume service contract to attract GP referrals, appropriateness of GP referrals for a directly-managed hospital).
- Those reflecting aspects of service design and delivery which market research has shown to be difficult to achieve (e.g. reducing lengths of NHS waiting lists and waiting time from GP referral to first hospital appointment).
- Aspects of service where the NHS organization faces severe competitive pressure (e.g. flexibility of booking arrangements for cold surgery).
- Events or aspects of service likely to have a large effect on the NHS organization's public image (e.g. ambulance response to major accidents).
- Outcome, iatrogenesis, invasiveness, other side-effects, risks and social acceptability are critical in assessing pilot or experimental forms of service, followed by its capacity to contribute to the business plan, quality specification and service contract objectives.

Table 6.2 Critical tracking variables; a worked example from social care services for people with learning difficulties

1   Percentage of responses to referrals within 24 hours of referral (optimum level 100%).

2   Percentage of clients receiving services outside the locality (a proxy indicator of how comprehensive services are).

3   Percentage of clients receiving individual programme planning (optimum level 100%).

4   Realization of the 'five achievements': community presence, respect, choice, competencies and relationships (tracked using the appropriate outcome indicators).

5   Percentage of clients receiving segregated day care services (a proxy indicator for normalization; optimum level 0%).

6   Existence of policy and procedure for self- or citizen-advocacy, supplemented by checks on how the policy and procedure are implemented.

7   Tenancy status of clients (to indicate continuity and security of housing).

8   Availability of support services, monitored through audit of referrals to other agencies, service deficiencies revealed through audit of IPPs, internal care audit.

9   Existence of a complaints procedure and its ability to generate remedies, monitored through an audit of complaints.

10 Clients have a personal cash income large enough to meet their daily living needs (optimal level 100%).

11 Percentage of clients in residential care (optimum 0%).

12 Percentage of clients in residences with more than four clients (optimum 0%).

13 Percentage of clients in segregated short-term care (optimum 0%).

- Scale and direction of changes in public or user behaviour, in the case of promotional work. A critical tracking variable here is whether unhealthy behaviour has been prevented, or only deflected into a new channel (e.g. if anti-heroin activity succeeds mainly in diverting potential drug abusers to other drugs) or whether the promotion has even been counterproductive (e.g. by arousing children's curiosity about drugs not deterring abuse).
- Aspects of curing or caring services likely to have far-reaching consequences for patients. Health outcomes, iatrogenesis and the clinical and social quality of care are critical here. Table 6.2 illustrates such tracking variables with an example from social care of people with learning difficulties.

The purpose of tracking is to trigger corrective action or stimulate the raising of quality standards and the redesign of services. So in all cases (not only in monitoring service contracts) it is necessary to define both the target levels of the tracking variables and what levels of the tracking variables or what changes would trigger a response. If possible these levels, and the mechanism for initiating a response, should be agreed between clinicians, managers and other interested parties before tracking begins. Examples of events triggering a response might include:

- Falls over 5% in one quarter in referrals to the hospital from one general practice (or from all the GPs).
- A long-term rise in referrals not covered by a service contract.
- A promotional counterblast by the food industry or some other target for intersectoral planning.
- Rises of over 10% in avoidable factors in peri-operative deaths over a month.

The responses which such events could trigger are considered at step 24.

Periodicity

Practical considerations in deciding the frequency of market research are discussed in chapter 4 (step A, p. 82). However collection of tracking data must become a frequent routine if tracking is to serve its purposes. For critical and unstable variables such as hospital cross-infection control during outbreaks of infection or blood donations during periods of peak demand, weekly or even daily tracking might not be excessive.

Step 23. Decide data collection methods, collect and process data

Given the purposes, frequency, scale and possible commercial or political sensitivity of tracking data, most tracking data will normally have to be collected and analysed by the NHS organization itself. These considerations will, in practice, often provide the biggest single impetus to NHS organizations setting up the sort of market research infrastructure described in

Chapter 4, p. 108. Tracking has therefore to be the responsibility of the marketing manager, quality assurance co-ordinator or whoever else heads the marketing and market research infrastructure, but as always done on behalf of the service's line manager or clinicians. However internal tracking will have to be supplemented by tracking by external bodies when:

- Service contracts are operating; then the buyer will also track the seller's marketing (and other) performance in addition to the buyer and seller each internally tracking their own marketing activities. This also applies to FHSA tracking of general practices' activities.
- GPs adopt practice budgets, giving them a financial motive to track hospitals' performance, by the methods discussed below, as well as their own.
- Statutory bodies such as CHCs exercise their duties of independent scrutiny of the services.
- The RHA, or another third party, adjudicates disputes between buyers and sellers.
- Independent evaluation of services is required for accreditation, research or licensing purposes. (DHAs might reasonably make this a condition for licensing private nursing homes.) Service contracts could conceivably stipulate third-party tracking of services, for instance the external clinical audit of SGTs' services.

Methods for conducting the tracking research are as described in Chapter 4. For minor, day-to-day operational monitoring, informal methods ('management by walking about') will often suffice. More formal data collection methods for tracking will tend to be closed, structured and leading; for instance using observation checklists, administrative data and closed-question questionnaires. This is because the tracking variables are pre-determined as described above; there is less necessity here to seek previously unsuspected areas for management intervention. How much detail is required depends upon how many tracking variables are selected, and upon whether 'trigger' levels have been reached. Tracking data is summary in normal circumstances ('broad' rather than 'deep', in the language of Chapter 4) until trigger levels are passed. Then one possible response is to track the problematic variables in closer detail (see step 24, p. 165).

The main practical problem in handling tracking data is its sheer quantity. One solution is not to track all wards, departments and other services perpetually but to track aggregate, summary data continuously and then rotate the collection of more detailed tracking data among the wards and departments. Vignette 6.2 illustrates how one outpatients department did this.

External tracking is likeliest to be revealing, and to motivate the maintenance of prescribed service standards, when it is conducted either without prior warning, or through rights of access to all patients, premises and records (not just those made available by mutual *ad hoc* arrangement).

However one method of health service market research is especially

---

Vignette 6.2   Tracking out-patient services

After undertaking market research, managers at Stafford DGH had identified areas for improving out-patient services. These included reviewing the working system, producing a new patient handbook, revising hospital signs and reaching agreement with staff on acceptable standards for patient waiting times. It was agreed to investigate whether there should be new forms of staff induction and consumer relations training. The manager responsible for out-patients helped formulate how the effects of implementing these charges would be tracked.

The original market research methods had included a questionnaire to staff and patients and it was decided to re-issue this at six-monthly intervals as a tracking tool. Because 30 clinics were involved it was decided to stagger their tracking cycles. Thus tracking data on the orthopaedics and paediatrics clinics would be collected during the eighth week after presentation of tracking data on the first clinics to have been tracked; general medicine and rheumatology clinic tracking data would be collected 16 weeks afterwards and so on until all the clinics were reviewed. The cycle would then be repeated. This method made the flow of incoming questionnaires more even and more manageable as a routine. The possibility of using routinely collected PAS data to monitor patient waiting times at clinics was also considered; but the obstacle here was the difficulty in modifying the PAS computer software for the purpose. Reports on the tracking results were to be synchronized with UMT meetings in such a way that each UMT meeting considered results on five questionnaire questions, gradually working through the questionnaire topics in cyclical fashion.

---

suited for clinical tracking. It also deserves closer attention because the Department of Health appears to support it as a major vehicle for carrying quality assurance into the clinical domain. Clinical audit is now spreading from the US into the NHS, and from medicine into nursing and other health professions. For NHS GPs the corresponding process is the clinical or service audit of patients recently discharged from hospital. In introducing it to NHS services the following decisions have to be made:

- What should the range of the audit be? Medical audit can be conducted within a single consultant 'firm', across a speciality or group of related specialities (e.g. general surgery with plastic surgery and orthopaedics) or can extend beyond the medical professions to cover the whole clinical episode (i.e. all clinical aspects of the quality chain).[17]
- Clinical audit is usually carried out internally to the hospital or general practice but there is no reason in principle why cases cannot be reviewed by an external clinical peer.
- What is to be done to safeguard confidentiality and who may have access to the results. One solution is to anonymize the medical record in regard to the patient; this protection may also be extended to the practitioners. It is

to summary results in this form that NHS managers and marketers are likeliest to be able to negotiate access with the clinical professions.

- Whether and how to organize different levels of audit. A common US model begins audit with an initial screening of medical records by a nurse practitioner or medical records officer. All records exhibiting defined events (e.g. maladministration of drugs or a patient complaint), plus a random selection of the others, then undergo internal peer review by an internal audit committee. The latter may then refer controversial cases, or cases satisfying further predetermined criteria (e.g. *prima facie* evidence of malpractice), to an external peer review.
- Which models of clinical audit to pursue. Other European variants may prove more useful models for the NHS because in the US system clinical audit has a largely defensive function of minimizing the risk of malpractice litigation.

Many existing clinical management activities can contribute to audit. The Netherlands National Quality Assurance proposals suggest the inclusion of the daily clinical rounds, X-ray meetings, referral meetings and the daily report, and of the periodic accident, drugs and ethical committees' meetings, autopsy meetings, infection control meetings. In the Netherlands medical audits are regularly carried out on anti-coagulant, antibiotics, blood transfusions, infusion and bladder catheterization policies, on pre-operative assessments, pressure sore incidence and medical record keeping.[18] In the NHS, follow-up clinics have provided an easy vehicle for clinical tracking but such clinics are gradually decreasing under pressure of resource constraints and waiting lists.

How NHS staff are likely to react to the approaching introduction of clinical audit is a very under-researched area. Recent market research by the Manchester Health Services Management Unit suggests that clinical audit is most likely to be acceptable to nurses when it:

- Is applied in a flexible, non-authoritarian way.
- Emanates from the nursing profession itself.
- Allows for local difficulties in care delivery, such as over-work and understaffing.
- Allows nurses to add local targets and standards to NHS-wide standards.
- Allows nurses to interpret, qualify or explain aberrant results.
- Is used to defend and improve existing standards of care not police or penalize individual nurses' work.
- Explains and interpret the results of audit, not simply gives a 'pass or fail' result.
- Accommodates the particular clinical audit interests of specialties such as midwifery and health visiting within the broad nursing profession.

Since NHS nurses have tended to follow the medical role model in professionalizing themselves, as have other NHS paramedical professions, these findings may also apply to other NHS clinicians. That conclusion must, however, be tentative pending further research.

Step 24. Select feedback route, present data and decide response

The point of tracking is to stimulate action to improve services, communications or profits. So the main principle in feeding back tracking data is to ensure that the results reach above all the managers or clinicians responsible for the impact of the service being tracked and those who have power to initiate remedial action. The feedback route required in each case therefore depends on what variables are being tracked.

Operational tracking results on the day-to-day implementation of marketing activity within the hospital or general practice have to be fed back to line managers, supervisors and clinicians. A US model is for tracking data to be fed back monthly to each departmental meeting. The meeting notes any problems occurring, the action to be taken and, at a later meeting, the results. Normally this feeds back into a review and modification of steps 17 to 21B (pp. 124–59). Evaluative tracking of experimental or pilot schemes for new service design also falls into this category, and has also to be fed back to the applied researchers.

Promotional tracking of the impact of NHS communications on target audiences' beliefs and attitude has to be fed back to line managers and clinicians (on operational promotions), to health education and promotion staff (on health promotion and intersectoral promotions) and to general managers (on public image and health policy matters). Review and modification of steps 17 to 21A (pp. 124–42) would be the normal consequence.

Tracking results on compliance with service contracts have to reach the contract managers on both the SGT and the buyer sides, and GPs in practices with practice budgets. In the short term these results normally trigger much the same responses as operational tracking (modifying steps 17 to 21B: and see below), in the longer term they inform the periodic renegotiation of the service contract (beginning at step 6 or even step 1).

Summary tracking data on strategic objectives have to be fed to general managers, the Health Authority or SGT Directorate or RHA or Department of Health (depending on circumstances) with detailed data going to the financial departments, directors of public health (in the case of buyers), and business planners. Normally this will inform the periodic review of the prime objectives and business plan (steps 1 and 6).

Analytic and presentational requirements for market research in general (with tracking as an instance) are outlined in Chapter 4. For tracking purposes time-series, comparisons with business plan objectives and (for sellers) comparison with competitors' performance are especially necessary.

The appropriate feedback route also depends on what response is likely to be required; the more serious the response likely to be required, the more senior the manager or clinician that the tracking results must be reported to.

The responses which might be triggered by tracking results can be listed in increasing order of seriousness and decreasing order of frequency:

- More detailed evaluation or investigation, e.g. to ascertain causes of an increase in drug abuse, NAI reports or cross infection.
- Managerial intervention, for instance to adjust the staffing, rewards, building or maintenance schemes or service design. For clinicians the corresponding level of response would be to adjust treatment plans or protocols, or referral patterns. Where several clinicians are involved, informal discussions are sometimes used, including informal discussions between consultants and GPs over changes in GP referral patterns and the reason for this. These first two events are common, routine responses to operational tracking results.
- A promotional response, for example in reply to public or media criticism, or developing alternative promotional media. Publication of tracking data itself can be a means of instigating action as the furore following publication of US hospital mortality rates showed. The nearest NHS equivalent are the publication of waiting list and beddage data by John Yates and others,[19] and the occasional appearance of summary data from CEPOD and the corresponding maternity inquiry.
- In the case of service contracts, RHAs or even the Department of Health may be able to adjudicate over responsibility and liability for failures to satisfy the contract.
- Sanctions are theoretically available in case of serious failure to comply with the service contract. However buyers who withhold large cash payments risk disrupting existing patient services and hence of harming patients unless payments for service contracts have been structured (like some building contracts) so that the profit element can be distinguished from the wages, salary and other production cost elements. For a seller the obvious defence will be to claim that they have simply fulfilled the service contract as drafted (or misdrafted). The availability of sanctions thus depends on the buyer's skill in drafting a service specification and service contract (steps 10 and 15 pp. 69 and 122).
- As a last resort it is possible, although practically disruptive, to suspend a service, a provider, promotional work or a service contract (this already happens in the event of industrial action, allegation of professional misconduct or major accident). This would lead to modification of service specification or contract renegotiation.

After tracking the NHS marketing cycle has to be repeated, starting at steps 1, 6, or 17 as the case may be.

Postscript

Marketing, internal markets and health service structure

Previous chapters show how marketing for commercialized health service providers such as NHS Self-Governing Trusts differs from marketing in directly managed public sector health services and buying organizations. The difference lies not only in the marketing process (see steps 4 and 5 in Figure 3.1, step 13B in Figure 5.1) but, far more, in the substantive objectives served by marketing (see step 1, p. 46 above). It then takes concrete form in such matters as the mix of services offered (step 5, p. 53), their quality specifications step 10, p. 69) and their design (step 18B, p. 143). The difference is between the primacy of financial and the primacy of 'real' health objectives respectively.

In a health and social care system in transition from a directly managed, publicly funded model to an internal market these differences will be attenuated in the short term. Practical difficulties will reinforce sheer organizational inertia in adjusting to new, commercial imperatives, as NHS managers' overload in trying to implement *Working for Patients* during 1990 illustrates. A prudent government will also try so to implement internal markets so as to minimise the political and electoral costs of the reforms and their consequences. Yet insofar as internal markets live up to their name, these differences in health care organizations' objectives and activities will inevitably assert themselves in the longer term, making commercial and health objectives increasingly difficult to reconcile.

Whilst this book was written, implementation of an internal market for health care in Britain proceeded at accelerating pace. Insofar as NHS managers have discretion in how to implement these reforms, the question arises of what approach is likeliest to realize the potential benefits of health service marketing outlined at the end of chapter 2 (p. 39). Preceding chapters suggest that this is much likelier to occur through directly-managed services (or the nearest approximation that service contracting allows) than through commercialized, or semi-commercialized, SGTs. That SGTs will remain, for the moment, in public ownership makes little difference to this. For most consumers of health care the strongest arguments in favour of non-market, or failing that directly-managed, health services are marketing arguments.

References and notes

Chapter I

1 Department of Health (1989) *Working for Patients*, p. 39. London, HMSO.
2 Department of Health *Working for Patients*, p. 24.
3 E.g. Sheaff, R. (1989) *'A Most Far Reaching Reform': The Prime Minister's review of the NHS Examined*, Manchester, Health Services Management Unit Occasional Paper 69.
4 Sheaff, R. & O'Grady, E. (1989) *Consumerism, Marketing and Quality in the NHS. Some Lessons from other Organisations*, Bristol, NHS Training Authority.
5 E.g. Leneman, L., Jones, L. & Maclean, U. (1987) *Consumer Feedback for the NHS. A Literature Review*, London, Kings Fund.
6 Dixon, P. & Carr-Hill, R. (1989) *The NHS and its Customers iii Customer Feedback Surveys – A Review of Current Practice*, York, Centre for Health Economics.
7 E.g. Gough, I. (1984) *The Political Economy of the Welfare State*, London, Macmillan. O'Connor, J. (1973) *The Fiscal Crisis of the State*, New York, St Martins.
8 *Report of the Royal Commission on the National Health Service* (1979), pp. 9–12, London, HMSO.
9 Griffiths, R. (1988) *Community Care: Agenda for Action. A Report to the Secretary of State for Social Services*, London, HMSO.
10 WHO (1985) *Health for All by the Year 2000*, targets 27, 31, Geneva, WHO.
11 WHO (1986) *Evaluating the Success of Health For All 2000*, pp. 76–8, Copenhagen, WHO European Region.
12 Beveridge, W. (1942) *Social Insurance and Allied Services*, pp. 6, 9, London, HMSO Cmnd. 6404.
13 Hansard, 30th April 1946.
14 *Working for Patients* endorses this.
15 Department of Health and Social Security (1980) *Inequalities in Health*, London, DHSS.
16 E.g. Doyal, L. & Gough, I. (1984) 'Theory of Human Needs', *Critical Social Policy*, 10, 6–38.
17 Ibid.
18 E.g. Sheaff, R. (1988) 'Needs and Justice in Health Resource Allocation', in Fairbairn, G. and Fairbairn, S. (eds) *Ethical Issues in Caring*, p. 119, Aldershot, Avebury.
19 Jackson, P. M. (1987) 'Value for money: whose money is it anyway?' in National Consumer Council (ed.) *Performance Measurement and the Consumer*, p. 38, London, NCC.

20 Kotler P. & Zaltman G. (1971) 'Social marketing: an approach to planned social change' *Journal of Marketing*, **35**, 55, 69. Kotler, P. & Levy, S. J. (1969) 'Broadening the Concept of Marketing' *Journal of Marketing*, **33** 10–15.

21 Griffiths, R. (1983) Letter to Norman Fowler of 6 October 1983, (the first Griffiths 'Report') p. 9.

22 *Working for Patients*, pp. 6–7, Brindle, D., 'Hospitals to raise funds with Chablis and manicures', *Guardian*, 12 September 1990, p. 20.

23 E.g. Evans, J. R. & Berman, B. (1987) *Marketing*, London, Macmillan. Stanton, W. (1981) *Fundamentals of Marketing*, London, McGraw Hill. Zikmund, W. & D'Amico, M. (1984) *Marketing*, Chichester, Wiley.

24 Evans & Berman, *Marketing*, p. 69.

25 Kotler & Levy 'What Consumerism Means for Marketers' p. 15.

26 Boston Consulting Group (1968) *Perspectives on Experience*, Boston, BCG.

27 Ansoff H. I. (1957) 'Strategies for diversification' *Harvard Business Review*, (Sept/Oct 1957) **25**, 113–124.

28 Phillips L. W., Chang B. R. & Buzzell, R. D. (1983) 'Product quality, cost positions and business performance. A test of some key hypotheses' *Journal of Marketing*, **47** (2) 26–443.

29 Lubatkin, M. & Pitts, M. (1983) 'PIMS: fact or folklore?' *Journal of Business Strategy*, **3** (3) 38–43.

30 Porter M. E. (1980) *Competitive Strategies: Techniques for Analysing Industries and Competition*, New York, Free Press.

31 Kotler, P. & Clarke, R. (1987) *Marketing for Health Care Organisations*, ch. 4, London, Prentice Hall.

32 Stapleton, J. (1981) 'Making a marketing plan' in Rines, M. (ed.) *Marketing Handbook*, Aldershot, Gower.

33 E.g. Crump M. (1985) *The Marketing Research Process*, Englewood Cliffs, Prentice Hall. Chisnall, P. (1975) *Marketing. A Behavioural Analysis*, London, McGraw Hill. Prince, M. (1982) *Consumer Research for Management Decisions*, Chichester, Wiley.

34 Cf. Prince *Consumer Research for Management Decisions*, pp. 47–60, 91.

35 References can be found in the better-researched marketing texts e.g. Chisnall's *Marketing. A Behavioural Analysis* and Evans and Bermans's *Marketing*.

36 Haley, R. C. (1968) 'Benefit segmentation. A decision-oriented research tool' *Journal of Marketing* **32**, 30–35. Thomas, M. (1980) 'Market segmentation' *Quarterly Review of Marketing*, Autumn, pp. 25–8.

37 E.g. Leiss, W., Kline, S. & Jhally, S. (1986) *Social Communication in Advertising*, London, Methuen. Festinger, L. (1962) *A Theory of Cognitive Dissonance*, London, Tavistock. Dyer, G. (1982) *Advertising as Communication*, London, Nelson.

38 Cf. Yankelovich, D. (1964) 'New criteria for market segmentation' *Harvard Business Review* **42**, 83–90, Crump, M. (1985) *The Marketing Research Process*, chp. 6, pp. 102–124, Englewood Cliffs, Prentice Hall.

39 Stapleton 'Making a Marketing Plan', p. 103.

40 McCarthy, E. J. (1978) *Basic Marketing: A Managerial Approach*, Homewood, Irwin.

41 Britt, S. H. & Boyd, H. W. (eds) (1968) *Marketing Management and Administration*, p. 315, New York, McGraw Hill.

42 Britt & Boyd *Marketing Management And Administration*, p. 96. Chisnall, *Marketing. A Behavioural Analysis*, p. 156.

43 Packard, V. (1961) *The Waste Makers*, pp. 55, 58. London, Longman.

44 E.g. Leiss, W. Kline, S. & Jhally, S. *Social Communication in Advertising*.

45 British Standards Institute *BS 5750: 1979 Quality Systems*; & see chapter 4, pp. 80f.

46 Kotler & Clarke *Marketing for Health Care Organisations*, p. 21.

47 Widgery, D. (1979) *Health in Danger*, p. 86. London, Macmillan.
48 'Market Forces' BBC radio 4 9th February 1989.
49 *Which*, August 1989.
50 Packard, V. (1981) *The Hidden Persuaders*, p. 15. Harmondsworth, Penguin.
51 Taylor, P. (1984) *The Smoke Ring*, pp. 133f, London, Sphere.
52 Packard, *The Hidden Persuaders*, pp. 148–150.
53 Williams, R. C. (1985) 'Sales: Evaluating the Plan', in Paul D. T. (ed.) *Building Marketing Effectiveness in Healthcare*, p. 21, Chicago, American Marketing Association.
54 As a starting point; Argyle, M. (1985) *The Social Psychology of Work*, chp. 9, Harmondsworth, Penguin. Handy, C. (1981) *Understanding Organisations*, Harmondsworth, Penguin. Herzberg, F. (1968) 'One More Time; How do you Motivate Employees?' *Harvard Business Review*, **46**, 53–62.
55 American Marketing Association, Conference Proceedings, 1960. The AMA replaced this definition in 1985.
56 Kotler & Clarke, *Marketing for Health Care Organisations*, pp. 5–6. Kotler, P. (1972) 'A generic concept of marketing' *Journal of Marketing*, **36**, 49.
57 Kotler 'A Generic Concept of Marketing', pp. 49–50.
58 E.g. Hunt, R. (1983) *Marketing Theory. The Philosophy of Marketing Science*, chp. 1, Homewood, Irwin.

Chapter 2

1 Compare the American Marketing Association's view cited in chapter 1.
2 Packard, V. (1981) *The Hidden Persuaders*, pp. 200–203, Harmondsworth, Penguin. Haller, T. (1983) *Danger: Marketing Research at Work*, p. 3, Westport, Quorum.
3 Klein, R. (1983) *The Politics of the National Health Service*, p. 153, Harlow, Longman.
4 Butler, J. R. & Vaile, M. S. B. (1984) *Health and Health Services. An Introduction to Health Care in Britain*, p. 95, London, RKP. Klein, R. *Complaints Against Doctors. A Study in Professional Accountability*, p. 7.
5 Klein, R. (1975) *Complaints Against Doctors*, p. 153. London, Charles Knight.
6 Klein, R. (1983) *The Politics of the National Health Service*, p. 153, Harlow, Longman.
7 Leonard-Barton, D. (1981) 'Professionals as "information priests" in the diffusion of innovations: the case of dentists', in Bloom, P. N. (ed.) *Consumerism and Beyond. Perspectives on the Future Social Environment*, p. 124. Massachusetts, Marketing Science Institute.
8 Cang, S. (1978) 'Structural analysis of doctor–patient relationships', in Jaques, E. (ed.) *Health Services. Their Nature and Organisation and the role of Patients, Doctors and the Health Professions*, p. 67, London, Heinemann.
9 Kotler & Clarke, *Marketing for Health Care Organisations*, p. 369.
10 Pollitt, C. (1987) 'Performance measurement and the consumer: hijacking a bandwagon', in National Consumer Council (ed.) *Performance Measurement and the Consumer*, p. 47, London, NCC.
11 Cang, S. (1978) 'Structural Analysis of the Doctor–Patient Relationship' in Jaques, E. (ed.) (1978) *Health Services*, p. 67, London, Heinemann.
12 Packard, *The Hidden Persuaders*, pp. 66f, 75f, 92f, 99f, 112f.
13 Debate on the NHS Bill, April 1946.
14 Packard, *The Hidden Persauders*, p. 235.
15 Griffith, B., Rayner, G. & Mohan, J. (1985) *Commercial Medicine in London*, London, GLC.

16 Cartwright, A. (1967) *Patients and Their Doctors*, p. 22, London, RKP.

17 Taylor, P. (1985) *The Smoke Ring*, pp. 180–181 (original emphases), London, Sphere.

18 Culyer, A. J. (1987) 'The future of health economics in the UK' in Teeling-Smith, G. (ed.) *Health Economics: Prospects for the Future*, p. 21, London, OHE.

19 Culyer A. J. (1976) *Need and the National Health Service. Economics and Social Choice*, p. 180, London, Martin Robinson.

20 Cf. Kohn, R. (1983) *The Health Centre Concept in Primary Health Care*, p. 48, Copenhagen, WHO European Region.

21 British Medical Association (1981) *The Handbook of Medical Ethics*, pp. 51, 54, 56–57, London, BMA.

22 Data from Heald G. & Wybrow, R. J. (1985), *The Gallup Survey of Britain*, pp. 74, 258, London, Croom Helm.

23 Illich, I. (1977) *Medical Nemesis*, Harmondsworth, Penguin.

24 *Pace*, Tolliday, H. 'Clinical autonomy', in Jaques, E. (ed.) (1978) *Health Services*, p. 25, London, Heinemann.

25 Cf. Higgins, J. (1988) on the avoidance of waiting lists, in *The Business of Medicine*, pp. 172–3, Basingstoke, Macmillan.

26 For examples cf. Barrowcliffe, M. (1989) 'Managers will tie GPs' hands' *Medeconomics*, **10** (6), 84–85 and Slingsby, C. (1989) 'Will you bow to peer group pressure?', *Medeconomics*, **10** (5), 44.

27 Daniels, N. (1981) 'Health care needs and distributive justice', *Philosophy and Public Affairs*, (Spring) **10** (2), 153, 158.

28 Ibid. p. 158.

29 Ibid. pp. 160–161, 172–174.

30 Ibid. pp. 174–175.

31 Titmuss, R. (1970) *The Gift Relationship. From Human Blood to Social Policy*, p. 158, London, Allen & Unwin.

32 Ibid. pp. 144–157.

33 Ibid. pp. 245–246.

34 Widgery, D. (1979) *Health in Danger. The Crisis in the National Health Service*, p. 88, London, Macmillan.

35 *Which*, August 1989, p. 361.

36 Cf. *Which*, August, 1989 p. 405.

37 Kotler & Clarke, *Marketing for Health Care Organisations*, p. 27.

38 Packard, *The Hidden Persuaders*, p. 230.

39 *Ideal Home*, June 1989, p. 71.

40 *Looks* **47** August 1989, p. 38. Packard, *The Hidden Persuaders*, p. 230.

41 Kotler & Clarke, *Marketing for Health Care Organisations*, p. 431.

42 Interviewee, 'Market Forces', BBC radio 4, 9th February 1989.

43 Packard, *The Hidden Persuaders*, pp. 135f, 237.

44 Packard, *The Waste Makers*, pp. 55f, 68f.

45 Packard, *The Waste Makers*, p. 95.

46 Kotler & Clarke, *Marketing for Health Care Organisations*, p. 23.

47 Cf. Klein, *The Politics of the National Health Service*, p. 158.

48 Duncan Nichol's comments in the special edition of *NHS Management Executive News* of July 1990 seem to be targeted partly against this sort of objection.

49 Central Statistical Office (1989) *Social Trends 19*, p. 132, London, HMSO.

50 DHSS (1988) *Comparing Health Authorities*, p. 29, London, DHSS. OHE (1987) *Compendium of Health Statistics 1987*, fig. 3.34. London, OHE.

51 Butler J. R. & Vaile, M. S. B. (1984) *Health and Health Services*, p. 98, London, Routledge.

52 Heald and Wybrow, *The Gallup Survey of Britain*, pp. 127, 129, 131, 282: Klein, *The Politics of the National Health Service*, p. 125. Jowell, R., Witherspoon, S. and

Brook, L. (eds) (1987) *British Social Attitudes – the 1987 Report*, pp. 2, 16, Aldershot, Gower. See also p. 41 of the 1989 report by the same editors and publisher.

53 Concern over this prompted such publications as; Institute of Health Services Management (1988) *Alternative Delivery and Funding of Health Services*, London, IHSM.

54 E.g. *The Pattern of the In-Patient's Day*, (1958) London, HMSO. *The Welfare of Children in Hospital*, (1959) London, HMSO.

55 E.g. Kotler, P. (1975), *Marketing For Non-Profit Organisations*, Arlington, VTNC.

56 E.g. Stapleton, 'Making a Marketing Plan', p. 115.

57 E.g. Doyal, L. & Gough, I. 'A theory of human needs', *Critical Social Policy*; Sheaff, 'Needs and Justice in Health Resource Allocation', p. 119.

58 Groncoos, C. (1982) *Strategic Management and Marketing in the Service Sector*, p. 137, Helsingfors, Swedish School of Economic and Business Administration.

Chapter 3

1 Cf. Crosby, P. B. (1979) *Quality is Free*, pp. 36, 69, New York, McGraw Hill.

2 Donabedian, A. (1980) *The Definition of Quality and Approaches to its Assessment*, 1, 27, 79–85. Ann Arbor, Health Administration Press.

3 Maxwell, R. (1984) 'Quality assessment in health', *British Medical Journal*, (12 May). **288**, 1471.

4 British Standards Institute, *BS 4778*.

5 Crosby, *Quality is Free* pp. 9, 17, 127, 189, 267–8, 271, 292.

6 US Joint Commission on the Accreditation of Hospitals, Introduction to the accreditation manual, p. 8.

7 The concept of instrumental needs is discussed more fully in the ethical literature (e.g. Sheaff, 'Needs and Justice in Health Resource Allocation'. This definition implies that the BSI and Crosby definitions are potentially acceptable but under-defined, and the Maxwell and Donabedian definitions over-defined special cases, only valid if further research indicates that NHS users actually do want and need equity, adequate service documentation, etc.

8 *Working For Patients* and *Caring For Patients* give broad outlines, as do other national policy documents such as *Maternity Care in Action* and *Health for All 2000*.

9 Kotler & Clarke, *Marketing for Health Care Organisations*, p. 44.

10 Kotler & Clarke, *Marketing for Health Care Organisations*, pp. 44, 78.

11 BMA/Gallup poll, June 1989 *Health Services Journal*, **5159**, 844.

12 E.g. Cartwright, A. (1983) *Health Surveys in Practice and Potential: A Critical Review of their Scope and Methods*, London, Kings Fund. A useful summary of the indicators already collected in the UK is in Meredith Davies, J. B. (1983) *Community Health, Preventive Medicine and Social Services*, chp. 3 pp. 39–72, Eastbourne, Balliere Tindall.

13 Bayley, M., Seyd, R. & Tennant, A. (1989) *Local Health and Welfare: Is Partnership Possible? A Study of the Dinnington Project*, Basingstoke, Gower.

14 Neumann, B., Sheaff R. & Peel, V. (1990) *Costing Issues Arising from the Resource Management Initiative*, London, Department of Health (in press).

15 Porter M. E. (1985) *Competitive Advantage*, London, Macmillan. Porter M. E. (1980) *Competitive Strategies: Techniques for Analysing Industries and Competition*, New York, Free Press. Day, G. S. (1984) *Market Planning. The Pursuit of Competitive Advantages*, St Paul, West.

16 Cf. Higgins, J. (1988) *The Business of Medicine*, p. 95, Table 3.1, London, Macmillan.

17 E.g. Bush J. W., Chen, M. M. & Patrick, D. L. (1973) 'Health status index in cost

effectiveness: analysis of PKU program', in Berg, R. L. (ed) *Health Status Indexes*, p. 172, Chicago, Hospital Research and Education Trust. King P. 'The development of health indices' pp. 27–29; Kneppreth N. P., Gustafson, D. H., Rose, J. H. & Leifer, R. P. in Berg, op. cit. pp. 231–237. Rosser R. M. & Watts V. C. (1972) 'The measurement of hospital output', *International Journal of Epidemiology*, **1** (4), 361–368.

18 Atkinson, C. (1990) 'Creating Customer Driven Organisations; A Systemic Approach to Enhancing Quality and Profitability', seminar, University of Monterey.

19 *Working for Patients*, p. 7.

20 Brown, P. (1981) 'The mental patients' rights movement and mental health institutional change', *International Journal of Health Services*, **11** (4), 535.

21 'Ideological' in the technical sense defined by McClellan, D. (1986) *Ideology*, chp. 3, Milton Keynes, Open University Press.

22 McEwen, J. (1983) 'The Nottingham Health Profile: a measure of perceived health', in Teeling Smith, G. (ed) *Measuring the Social Benefits of Medicine*, p. 76, London, OHE.

23 Raynor, P. A. (1988) 'Severity measurement systems', *Health Care Competition Week*, 16 May, pp. 10–16.

24 Bergner, M., Bobbitt, R. A., Pollard, W. E., Martin, D. P. & Gillson, B. S. (1976) 'The sickness impact profile; validation of a health status measure', *Medical Care* **14** (1), 58–59.

25 Brooks, R. 'Health indicators in arthritis' in Teeling Smith, G. (ed) (1983) *Measuring the Social Benefits of Medicine*, p. 87, London, OHE.

26 E.g. Huskisson A. I. (1974) 'Measurement of pain', *Lancet*, **2**, 1127–1131.

27 See Culyer, A. J., Lavers, R. J. & Williams, A. (1972) 'Health indicators', in Shonfield A. & Shaw S. (ed) *Social Indicators and Social Policy*, pp. 102–103, London, Heinemann/SSRC. Culyer, A. J. (1976) *Need and the National Health Service*, London, Martin Robinson pp. 102f. Kind, P. 'The development of health indicators', in Teeling Smith (ed.) op. cit. p. 30.

28 Summarized in Raynes, N. V. (1988) *Annotated Directory of Measures of Environmental Quality for use in Residential Services for People with a Mental Handicap*, Manchester, Manchester University Department of Social Policy and Social Work.

29 Many further references are in Challis, D. J. (1981) 'Measurement of Outcome in Social Care of the Elderly', *Journal of Social Policy*, **10**, 179–208.

30 Isaacs, B. & Walkey F. A. (1963) 'The Mental Status Score', *American Journal of Psychiatry*, **120**, 173–174.

31 Cf Jennet, B. (1982) *High Technology Medicine. Benefits and Burdens*, p. 60 London, Nuffield Provincial Hospitals Trust.

32 Cf. Gillion, C., Schieber, G. & Poullier, J.-P. (1983) *Measuring Health Care 1960–1983. Expenditure, Costs and Performance*, p. 126, Paris, OECD.

33 World Health Organization (1985) *Health For All 2000*, appendices Geneva, WHO.

34 Raynes, N. V. (1988) *Annotated Directory of Measures of Environmental Quality for use in Residental Services for People with a Mental Handicap*, Manchester, Manchester University Department of Social Policy and Social Work.

35 E.g. the *Quality Assurance Abstracts* produced quarterly by the Department of Health and the Kings Fund.

36 Teeling-Smith, G. & Starfield, B. (1985) *The Effectiveness of Medical Care. Validating Clinical Wisdom*, Baltimore, Johns Hopkins UP. Shaw, C. (1986) *Introducing Quality Assurance*, pp. 22–23, London, Kings Fund. *Quality Assurance in Health Care* [journal], *Health Care Quality Assurance* [journal], *Quality Review Bulletin*, Chicago (US Joint Commission on Accreditation of Hospitals).

37 E.g. the isoquant analysis in the works by Williams and Culyer cited above.
38 House of Commons Social Services Committee (1980) *Perinatal and Neonatal Mortality*, London, HMSO.
39 The most obvious influence was Enthoven's (1985) *Reflections on the Management of the National Health Service. An American looks at Incentives and Efficiency in Health Services Management in the UK*, London, Nuffield Provincial Hospitals Trust.
40 Rosser, R. M. & Watts, V. C. (1972) 'The measurement of hospital ouput', *International Journal of Epidemiology*, **1** (4) 366, Fig. 6.
41 Williams, A. (1974) 'Measuring the effectivity of health care systems', *British Journal of Preventive and Social Medicine*, **28**, 198.
42 SDS database severity stage 2; unpublished SDS document.
43 E.g. in Rosser and Watts, *op. cit.*
44 Ibid.
45 E.g. Ratcliffe, J. W. & Gonzalez Della Valle, A. (1988) 'Rigour in health related research: towards an expanded conceptualisation', *International Journal of Health Services* **18** (3), 361–388. Rossi, P. H. & Freeman, R. E. (1982) *Evaluation: A Systematic Approach*, London, Sage. Bell, J. (1987) *Doing Your Own Research Project*, Milton Keynes, Open University Press.

Chapter 4

1 Heald G. & Wybrow R. J. (1985) *The Gallup Survey of Britain*, pp. 185–186, London, Croom Helm.
2 Contrast MacStravic, R. E. (1977) *Marketing Health Care*, p. 253, Germantown, Aspen.
3 E.g. Rossi, P. H. & Freeman, R. E. (1982) *Evaluation. A Systematic Approach*, London, Sage. Illsley, *Professional or Public Health*, p. 116f. Ratcliffe et al. (1983) 'Rigor in health related research: towards an expanded conceptualisation', International Journal of Health Services, (1988) **18** (3) 361–99. Holland, W. W. (ed) *Evaluation of Health Care*, Oxford, (Oxford University Press/EEC). Crane, J. A. (1982) *The Evaluation of Social Policies*, London, Kluwer Nijhoff. Kaluzny, A. D. & Veney, J. L. (1980) *Health Service Organisations: A Guide to Research and Assessment*, California. Milne, D. (1987) *Evaluating Mental Health Practice; Methods and Applications*, London, Croom Helm.
4 Caple, T. & Deighan, Y. (1986) *Managing Customer Relations. Taking A Snapshot*, London, North West Thames Regional Health Authority.
5 Nightingale, M. 'The hospitality industry: defining quality for a quality assurance programme – A study of perceptions', in Moores, B. (ed) (1986) *Are They Being Served?*, p. 14, Oxford, Philip Allan.
6 The idea was popularized by Peters, T. J. & Waterman, R. H. (1982) *In Search of Excellence. Lessons from America's Best-Run Companies*, pp. 122, 218f, New York, Harper & Row.
7 Department of Health (1989) *Homes are for Living In*, London, HMSO.
8 Cf. Katz, S., Akpom, C. A., Papsidero, J. A. & Weiss, S. T. (1973) 'Measuring the health status of populations' in Berg (ed) *Health Status Indicators*, p. 41. Fry, J. (1974) *Common Diseases: Their Nature Incidence and Care*, MPT.
9 E.g. National Association for the Welfare of Children in Hospital (1988) *Parents Staying Overnight in Hospital with their Children*, pp. 20f, London.
10 Dixon, P. & Carr-Hill R. (1989) *The NHS and its Customer iii Customer Feedback Surveys – A review of Current Practice*, York, Centre for Health Economics.
11 Dixon, P. & Carr-Hill, R. (1989) *The NHS and its Customer iii Customer Feedback Surveys – A review of Current Practice*, p. 9, York, Centre for Health Economics.

12 E.g. Luck, M., Lawrence, B., Pocock, B. and Reilly, K. (1988) *Consumer and Market Research in Health Care*, London, Chapman Hall. Fink, A. & Kosecoff, J. (1985) *How to Conduct Surveys. A Step by Step Guide*, Beverly Hills, Sage. Dixon, P. & Carr-Hill, R. (1989) *The NHS and Its Customers ii Customer Feedback Surveys – An introduction to Survey Methods*, York, Centre for Health Economics. Bell, J. (1987) *Doing Your Own Research Project*, Milton Keynes, Open UP. Prince (1982) *Consumer Research for Management Decisions*, Chichester, Wiley. Chisnall, P. (1975) *Marketing, A Behavioural Analysis*, London, McGraw Hill. Worcester, R. M. & Downham, R. J. (eds) (1978) *Consumer Market Research Handbook*, Wokingham, Van Nostrand Reinhold. Crump, M. (1985) *The Marketing Research Process*, Englewood Cliffs, Prentice Hall.

13 Heald, G. & Wybrow, R. J. (1985) *The Gallup Survey of Britain*, p. 287, London, Croom Helm.

14 Warren, M. (1986) 'Consumers' Association: which? why and how', in Moores, B. (ed) *Are They Being Served?*, p. 247, Oxford, Philip Allen.

15 Britt, S. H. & Boyd, H. W. (1968) *Marketing Management And Administration*, p. 414, New York, McGraw Hill. MacStravic, *Marketing Health Care*, p. 90, Germantown, Aspen.

16 MacStravic, R. E. (1977) *Marketing Health Care*, p. 285, Germantown, Aspen, in Teeling-Smith, G. (ed.) (1983) *Measuring the Social Benefits of Medicine*, London, Office of Health Economics.

17 Hunt, S. (1983) 'Measuring Health in Clinical Care and Clinical Trails', p. 16.

18 See note 3, p. 174.

19 See note 12, above.

20 Dixon, P. & Carr-Hill, R. (1989) *The NHS and its Customer iii Customer Feedback Surveys – A review of Current Practice*, p. 41, York, Centre for Health Economics.

21 Heald, G. & Wybrow, R. J. (1985) *The Gallup Survey of Britain*, p. 299, London, Croom Helm.

22 E.g. Gardner, G. (1978) *Social Surveys for Social Planners*, Milton Keynes, Open University Press.

23 Dixon, P. & Carr-Hill, R. (1989 *The NHS and its customers ii Customer Feedback Surveys – An Introduction to Survey Methods*, p. 21, York, Centre for Health Economics. p. 21.

24 Rose, M. (1984) *Industrial Behaviour. Theoretical Development Since Taylor*, Harmondsworth, Penguin.

25 McKeown, T. (1980) *The Role of Medicine*, pp. 19–20, London, NHPT.

26 Dixon, P. & Carr-Hill, R. (1989) *The NHS and its customers ii Customer Feedback Surveys – An Introduction to Survey Methods*, p. 29, York, Centre for Health Economics.

27 Packard, *The Hidden Persuaders*, p. 22.

28 Heath, A. (1986) 'Do people have consistent attitudes?', in Jowell R., Witherspoon S. & Brook L. (ed.) *British Social Attitudes. The 1986 Report*, p. 4, Aldershot, Gower.

29 Heald, G. & Wybrow, R. J. (1985) *The Gallup Survey of Britain*, p. 291. London, Croom Helm.

30 CASPE's Patsat System.

Chapter 5

1 McCarthy, E. J. (1978) *Basic Marketing. A Managerial Approach*, Homewood, Irwin.

2 See for instance Neumann, B., Sheaff R. & Peel, V. (1990) *Costing Issues Arising from the Resource management Initiative*, London, Department of Health (in press).

3 *Working for Patients* lists them as A&E, immediate hospital admissions from A&E, including much general surgery, general medicine, geriatrics, psychiatry, supporting OPD services. *Working for Patients*, p. 34.
4 NHS managers in personal correspondence with the writer.
5 *Working for Patients*, p. 34.
6 *Working for Patients*, p. 35.
7 Kotler & Clarke, *Marketing for Health Care Organisations*, p. 406.
8 Kotler & Clarke, *Marketing for Health Care Organisations*, p. 404.
9 E.g. Miller, R. B., Heiman, S. E. & Tuleja, T. (1986) *Strategic Selling*, New York, Warner. Fenton, J. (1984) *How to Sell Against Competition*, London, Heinemann.
10 Packard, *The Hidden Persuaders*, p. 46.
11 Chisnall, *Marketing. A Behavioural Analysis*, p. 239f.
12 Kolter & Clarke, *Marketing for Health Care Organisations*, pp. 517–518.
13 Kotler & Clarke, *Marketing for Health Care Organisations*, p. 507.
14 Packard, *The Hidden Persuaders*, p. 183.
15 Cf. Chisnall, *Marketing. A Behavioral Analysis*, p. 201.
16 I owe this point to David Baxter.
17 This is a standard behaviourist theme, e.g. in Skinner, B. F. (1973) *Beyond Freedom and Dignity*, Harmondsworth, Penguin.
18 Stern, A. (1990) 'Why AIDS ads need candour not cant' *Guardian*, 19th February p. 23.
19 BMA/Gallup poll, June 1989 *Health Services Journal*, 5159, p. 844; a confidential MORI poll of November 1989 reputedly reached similar conclusions.
20 Stern, A. (1990) 'Why AIDS ads need candour not cant', *Guardian*, 19th February p. 23.
21 Stocking, B. (1985) *Initiative and Inertia. Case Studies in the NHS*, London, NHPT.
22 Wadsworth, M. Butterfield, W. & Bloney, R. (1971) *Health and Sickness – The Choice of Treatment*, pp. 12–14, London, Tavistock.
23 Kotler & Clarke, *Marketing for Health Care Organisations*, p. 447.
24 Abelin, J., Brzezinski, Z. J. & Carstairs V. D. L. (eds) (1987) *Measurement in Health Promotion and Practice*, Copenhagen, WHO.
25 Stern, A. (1990) 'Why AIDS ads need candour not cant', *Guardian*, 19th February p. 23.
26 Judge K. (ed.) (1988) *Pricing the Social Services*, London, Macmillan.
27 Taylor, P. *The Smoke Ring*, p. 170–171 photograph).
28 Ibid. pp. 149–150.
29 Ibid. pp. 133–136.
30 Cf. Teeling-Smith, (ed.) *Measuring the Social Benefits of Medicine*, pp. 3–4, 165. Chapman et al., 'Why the Tobacco Industry Fears the Passive Smoking Issue', *International Journal of Health Services* (1990) **20** (3) 418.
31 E.g. Govoni, M., Eng, R. & Galper, M. (1986) 'Promotional mix', *Promotional Management*, p. 127f, Englewood Cliffs, Prentice Hall.
32 E.g. Hart, N. A. (1988) *Practical Advertising and Publicity*, London, Heinemann.
33 Silver, R. (ed.) (1985) *Health Service Public Relations. A Guide to Good Practice*, p. 28, London, Kings Fund.
34 E.g. the Brads and PIMS directories, published annually.
35 Silver, R. (ed.) (1985) *Health Service Public Relations*, p. 78, London, Kings Fund.
36 E.g. Leiss, W., Kline, S. & Jhally S. (1986) *Social Communication in Advertising*, London, Methuen.
37 An example is the current activity of the South Western RHA with the Line-Up consultancy.
38 Britt & Boyd, *Marketing Management and Administration*, p. 122.
39 Chisnall, *Marketing. A Behavioural Analysis*, pp. 183–184.

40 Cox, D. F. (1961) 'Clues for Advertising Strategists', *Harvard Business Review* **39**, 160–176.

Chapter 6

1 Donabedian, *The Definition of Quality and Approaches to its Assessment*, vol. i.
2 This is an argument for minimizing the number of procedures. Reliability can also be improved dramatically by duplicating procedures where possible (e.g. when the phlebotomist takes enough blood for a test to be repeated if necessary). The probability of two 97% reliable procedures both failing is only $(1-0.97)^2 = 0.09$ of 1%. For further details of the principles of risk management see the chapters by Disney and Rendell and by Keller, Sohal and Teasdale (1990) in Dale B. G. & Plunkett, T. J. (eds) *Managing Quality*, Hemel Hempstead, Phillip Allan.
3 Goffman, I. (1984) *Asylums. Essays on the Social Situation of Mental Patients and Other Inmates*, Harmondsworth, Penguin. passim.
4 Cartwright, A. (1967) *Patients and Their Doctors*, p. 181, London, RKP.
5 Traynor, J. 'The Local Authority Context' lecture, University of East Anglia, 17th July 1987.
6 Lewis, B. & Outram, M. (1986) 'Customer Satisfaction with Package Holidays' in Moore, B. (ed.) *Are They Being Served?*, p. 208, Oxford, Philip Allan.
7 Kotler & Clarke *Marketing for Health Care Organisations*, pp. 119, 123–124, 133–134. Chisnall, *Marketing. A Behavioural Analysis*, p. 155f.
8 E.g. Wall, A. (1990) *Ethics for Health Srvices Managers*, London, Kings Fund. Seedhouse, D. (1988) *Ethics, the Heart of Health Care*, Chichester, Wiley. Pappworth, M. H. (1967) *Human Guinea Pigs*, London, RKP.
9 See note 3 to chapter 4.
10 Inglis, B. (1981) *The Diseases of Civilization*, pp. 283–288, 193–298, St Albans, Granada.
11 This list adapts and extends Collard, R. (1989) *Total Quality*, London IPM, pp. 151–153, where a more detailed account of quality circles can also be found. See also Dale B. 'Experience with Quality Circle sand Quality Costs', in Moores (ed.) *Are They Being served?*, pp. 42, 45.
12 The term is borrowed from social policy studies. See Sabatier, P. & Mazmanian, D. (1979) 'Conditions of Effective Implementation; A Guide to Accomplishing Policy Objectives', *Policy Analysis* **iii** 481–483. Van Meter, D. & Van Horn, C. (1975) 'The Policy Implementation Process', *Administration and Society*, **vi**, 445–488. Webb, A. & Wistow, G. (1983) 'Public Expenditure and Policy Implementation: The Case of Community Care', *Public Administration* 1983 **lxi**, 21–44. Edelman, M. (1977) *Political Language. Words that Succeed and Policies that Fail*, New York, Academic Press. Majone, G. & Wildavsky, A. B. (1978) 'Implementation as Evolution', in Freeman, H. E. (ed.) *Policy Studies Annual Review*..
13 Hjern, B. & Porter, D. (1981) 'Implementation structures: new unit of administrative analysis', *Organisation Studies* **ii**, 211–227.
14 Liz Fox of Line-Up.
15 E.g. Collard, R. (1989) *Total Quality. Success Through People*, London, IPM.
16 O'Grady, E. W., in personal correspondance with the writer.
17 McConnachie, R. 'Medical Audit in North Derbyshire', lecture, NHS Studies Centre, Harrogate 31st March 1989.
18 Klazinga, N. 'Quality assurance in hospitals; should patients be able to influence?' Lecture, Manchester University, 11th January 1990.
19 Yates, J. M. (1982) *Hospital Beds. A Problem for Diagnosis and Management*, London, Heinemann.

Index